The Low Sugar Diet

Delicious recipes for clean eating

Robert V. Pelletier

Contents

ON RYE PIZZA

Chapter One

PESTO-BASED SAUSAGE SANDWICH

5 minutes to prepare – 10 minutes to cook • 2 herby Cumberland sausages, sliced lengthwise

• 1 ciabatta roll, sliced in half • 2 tablespoons fresh pesto • 1 jar roasted red pepper, sliced in half • 12 x 125g ball mozzarella, sliced DIRECTIONS 1.

Increase the temperature of the grill to high. Place the sausages cut-side down on a baking sheet and grill for 5-6 minutes, or until cooked through. Place the cut-side up ciabatta roll halves on a baking tray and spread pesto on each one. Grill for 2 minutes, or until golden and bubbling, on each half, with a pepper and mozzarella slice on top. Put the roll back together with the sausages and a handful of rocket, pressing firmly to keep the fillings in place.

Chapter Two

ROLLS OF AUBERGINE WITH SPINACH AND RICOTTA

ROLLS OF AUBERGINE WITH SPINACH AND RICOTTA

15 minutes to prepare - 45 minutes to cook - Provides food for INGREDIENTS: 4

• 2 aubergines, cut lengthwise into thin slices

• 2 tablespoons olive oil • 500 grams spinach • 250 grams tub ricotta • nutmeg grating • 350 grams jar tomato sauce • 4 tablespoons fresh breadcrumbs • 4 tablespoons parmesan (or vegetarian alternative)

DIRECTIONS

1st Step

Preheat the oven to 220 degrees Celsius/200 degrees Celsius fan/gas 7. Brush the aubergine slices with oil on both sides before placing them on a large baking sheet. Bake for 15-20 minutes, turning once, until tender.

Step 2 In the meantime, wilt the spinach in a large colander over a pot of boiling water. Allow to cool before squeezing out any excess water to ensure that it is completely dry. Combine the ricotta, nutmeg, and plenty of seasoning in a mixing bowl. Step 3 Spoon a spoonful of the cheesy spinach mixture into the center of each aubergine slice, fold over to form a parcel, and place in an ovenproof dish, sealed-side down. Pour tomato sauce over the top, top with breadcrumbs and cheese, and bake for 20-25 minutes, or until golden and hot.

Chapter Three

TART WITH MUSHROOM, RICOTTA, AND ROCKET

Prep: 10 mins - Cook: 25 mins - Provides food for 4
INGREDIENTS • 1 sheet ready-rolled puff pastry • 2 tbsp olive oil • 525g family pack mushroom, halved or quartered if large • 2 garlic cloves, 1 finely sliced, 1 crushed • 250g tub ricotta • good grating of nutmeg DIRECTIONS 1st Step

Heat oven to 220C/200C fan/gas 7 and place a baking sheet inside. Unroll the puff pastry onto a piece of baking parchment and score a 1.5cm border around the perimeter. Place the pastry on the baking sheet (still on the parchment) and bake for 10-15 minutes.

2nd Step

Meanwhile, heat the oil in a large lidded pan and cook the mushrooms for 2-3 minutes, stirring occasionally, while the pastry bakes. Remove the lid and add the sliced garlic, then cook for 1 min more to get rid of excess liquid.

3rd step

Season with salt and pepper after mixing the crushed garlic with the ricotta and nutmeg. Remove the puff pastry from the oven and gently press the risen center down. Spread over the ricotta mixture, then spoon on the mushrooms and garlic. Bake for 5 mins, then scatter over the parsley and rocket.

Chapter Four

RASPBERRY & LEMON POLENTA CAKE

Prep: 15 mins - Cook: 30 mins - Serves 8 INGREDIENTS

For the cake\s• 225g very soft butter\s• 225g caster sugar , plus 1 tbsp\s• 4 eggs , beaten

• 175g fine polenta\s• 50g plain flour\s• 1½ tsp baking powder\s• ½ tsp vanilla extract\s• finely grated zest of 1½ lemons\s• 200g frozen raspberry , left frozen\s• icing sugar , or more to taste (optional) (optional)

For the filling

• 100g soft cheese at room temperature (we used Philadelphia)\s• 1 tbsp icing sugar , or more to taste\s• finely grated zest of ½ lemon , plus a squeeze of juice\s• 142ml tub double cream\s• 100g frozen raspberry , defrosted

DIRECTIONS

1st Step

Heat oven to 190C/fan 170C/gas 5 and butter two 20cm sandwich tins. Line the bottom of the tins with baking paper. In a large bowl, beat the butter and 225g caster sugar together until creamy and light. Gradually add the egg, little by little, until all the egg is worked in and the mix is pale and fluffy. If the mix looks like it's starting to split, add 1 tsp of the flour, then carry on. Step 2\sPut the polenta in another bowl, then stir in the flour and baking powder. Beat the vanilla extract and zest into the eggy mix, then fold in the dry ingredients. Spoon half the batter into each tin and level the top. Scatter all but a handful of the raspberries over the mix and poke in gently.

Sprinkle one of the sponges with the 1 tbsp sugar. Bake for 20 mins until risen and golden, but still with a little wobble under the crust. Step 3\sOpen the oven, whip out the sugar-crusted sponge and quickly poke the remaining frozen raspberries into the top. Bake both sponges for 10 more mins or until springy in the middle. If this sounds too tricky, just leave the sponges to bake for 30 mins – the cake won't look as glam, but will still taste great (you can add the leftover berries to the filling instead) (you can add the leftover berries to the filling instead). Cool in the tin for 10 mins, then cool completely on a rack. Be careful when turning out the raspberry-topped sponge and slide it off its base rather than turning it upside down.

Step 4\sWhen the sponges are cold, beat the soft cheese with the icing sugar, lemon zest and a little of the juice to loosen if it needs it. Very lightly whip the cream so that it just holds its shape, then fold into the cheese. Fold in the defrosted raspberries. Use to sandwich the sponges together, sugar-crusted on top, and serve dusted with more icing sugar.

Chapter Five

PIZZA DOUGH

Prep: 15 mins plus rising (no cook) - Makes 4 pizzas INGREDIENTS\s• 500g '00' flour or plain flour, plus extra for dusting\s• 1 tsp salt\s• ½ tsp dried yeast (not fast-action)\s• 400ml warm water\s• oil, for greasing DIRECTIONS 1st Step

It's easiest to make this in a standing mixer with a dough hook (otherwise mix it in a bowl and knead on your work surface) (otherwise mix it in a bowl and knead on your work surface). Put the flour and salt in the bowl and mix the yeast into the water. It's always a good idea to wait 5 mins before using the liquid to see if the yeast is working – little bits will start to rise to the top and you'll know it's active.

Step 2\sTurn on the motor and pour in the liquid. Keep the speed on medium-high and it should come together as a ball. If the bottom is still sticking, tip in 1-2 tbsp of flour. Knead for 5-7 mins until the dough is shiny and it springs back when you press your finger into it. (If kneading by hand, it will take you about 10 mins.) Try not to add too much flour if you can. This is a slightly sticky dough, but that keeps it light and it rises beautifully.

Step 3\sUse oiled hands to remove the dough from the hook and bowl. Oil another bowl and place the dough in it. Turn it around so that it's lightly coated in the oil. Cover tightly with cling film and then a tea towel. Place in a draughtfree area that's warm and leave until the dough has doubled in size. If it's a hot day, it should only take 2 hrs to rise, but it could take 4 hrs if it's cold. (If you don't plan to use the dough for a day or two, place it in the fridge straight away; take it out 3-4 hrs before using. Punch it down first and bring it together on a floured surface.)

Step 4\sDivide the dough into 2 pieces for big pizzas or 4 for plate-sized ones, then shape into balls (see Shaping the dough in tips, below) – dust them in flour as they will be sticky. Keep them covered with a tea towel or cling film while you prepare the toppings. (you can also freeze them in sealed bags. Just thaw in the fridge on the day, then bring to room temperature 3 hrs before using.) Step 5\sTo shape the dough: If you want to get air pockets and a light but crisp dough, then don't use a rolling pin. It flattens and pops the air bubbles. (Two days in the fridge will produce the most air bubbles – take it out three to four hours before using.) If your dough is at room temperature, you can use your fingers to gently stretch the dough out. Once it's about 16cm, place the disc over the tops of your hands (not palm side) and use them to stretch it further, up to about 25cm. You can start pressing out the other discs, then wait to do the final bit when you're ready to cook.

Once you've mastered stretching the dough out, you can experiment with other shapes: rectangles, rounds or squares all look authentic.

Step 6\sTo cook the pizza: An outdoor gas barbecue is best for controlling the temperature, but charcoal

will give your pizza a more authentic, smoky flavour. For gas, turn the flames down to medium- low so that the bottom of the pizza doesn't burn. When cooking on a charcoal barbecue, let the coals turn grey before you pop on the pizza.

Step 7

Place the pizza on a floured baking sheet (with no edge) or a pizza peel – this is a flat pizza paddle with a long handle, which makes it easier to get the dough on and off the grill. The flour will provide the 'wheels' for it to slide onto the grill – don't use oil as it sticks more and won't transfer as well.

Step 8\sMake sure the grill is hot and the flames have died back if cooking on charcoal. Slide the dough onto the grill, close the lid (if your barbecue has one) and give it three to four minutes. The dough will puff up; it's ready when the bottom has light brown stripes. Use tongs to pull the dough off and turn it upside down. Step 9\sAssemble the pizza of your choice– see 'Goes well with', right, for topping suggestions. Remember that less is more, as the dough will stay crisper and the toppings will cook better. Step 10\sPlace the pizza back on the grill, uncooked-side down, and shut the lid. Give it another three to four minutes, then remove when the cheese is melted and the toppings are hot.

Chapter Six

ROASTED TOMATO, BASIL & PARMESAN QUICHE

Prep: 40 mins - Cook: 40 mins - Serves 8 INGREDIENTS

• 300g cherry tomato\s• drizzle olive oil\s• 50g parmesan (or vegetarian alternative), grated\s• 2 eggs\s• 284ml pot double cream\s• handful basil leaves, shredded, plus a few small ones left whole for scattering

For the pastry\s• 280g plain flour, plus extra for dusting\s• 140g cold butter, cut into pieces

DIRECTIONS

Step 1\sTo make the pastry, tip the flour and butter into a bowl, then rub together with your fingertips until completely mixed and crumbly. Add 8 tbsp cold water, then bring everything together with your hands until just combined. Roll into a ball and use straight away or chill for up to 2 days.

The pastry can also be frozen for up to a month.

Step 2\sRoll out the pastry on a lightly floured surface to a round about 5cm larger than a 25cm tin. Use your rolling pin to lift it up, then drape over the tart case so there is an overhang of pastry on the sides. Using a small ball of pastry scraps, push the pastry into the corners of the tin. Chill in the fridge or freezer for 20 mins. Heat oven to 200C/fan 180C/gas 6.

Step 3\sIn a small roasting tin, drizzle the tomatoes with olive oil and season with salt and pepper. Put the tomatoes in a low shelf of the oven.

Step 4\sLightly prick the base of the tart with a fork, line the tart case with a large circle of greaseproof paper or foil, then fill with baking beans. Blind-bake the tart for 20 mins, remove the paper and beans, then continue to cook for 5-10 mins until biscuit brown.

Step 5\sWhen you remove the tart case from the oven, take out the tomatoes, too.

Step 6\sWhile the tart is cooking, beat the eggs in a large bowl. Gradually add the cream, then stir in the basil and season. When the case is ready, sprinkle half the cheese over the base, scatter over the tomatoes, pour over the cream mix, then finally scatter over the rest of the cheese. Bake for 20- 25 mins until set and golden brown. Leave to cool in the case, cut the edges of the dough, then remove from the pan. Scatter over the remaining basil and serve in slices.

Chapter Seven

ROSEMARY CHICKEN WITH TOMATO SAUCE

Prep: 5 minutes - Cook: 30 mins - Provides food for 4
INGREDIENTS • 1 tablespoon olive oil • 8 boneless, skinless
chicken thighs • 1 rosemary sprig, finely chopped • 1 red
onion, finely sliced • 3 garlic cloves, sliced — 2 anchovy fillets,
diced • 400g can chopped tomatoes • 1 tablespoon capers,
drained • 75ml red wine (optional)

DIRECTIONS

Step 1 In a nonstick skillet, heat half the oil and brown the
chicken all over. Stir in half of the chopped rosemary and set
aside on a plate.

Step 2 Heat the remaining oil in the same pan, then gently sauté the onion for approximately 5 minutes, until tender. Fry for a few minutes more, until the garlic, anchovies, and remaining rosemary are aromatic. If using wine, pour it in with the tomatoes and capers, or 75ml water if without. Return the chicken pieces to the pan after bringing the water to a boil. Cook for 20 minutes, or until the chicken is cooked through. Season with salt and pepper and serve with crusty bread and a crisp green salad.

Chapter Eight

BROCCOLI & CHORIZO PENNE

Preparation time: 5 minutes; cooking time: 20 minutes - Provides food for • 400g penne • small head of broccoli, broken into small florets • 200g cooking chorizo, diced • 2 garlic cloves, crushed • 1 tbsp fennel seed • 200g low-fat cream cheese with garlic and herbs • parmesan and rocket leaves, to serve

DIRECTIONS

Step 1 Prepare the penne according to the package directions, adding the broccoli for the last 3 minutes. Drain, reserving a splash of the cooking water when done.

Step 2 In the meantime, in a large dry frying pan, fry the chorizo until it begins to turn golden and release its oils. Cook for an additional minute after adding the garlic and fennel seeds. Place the cooked penne in the pan with the chorizo. Stir in the cream cheese until it is completely melted, then add a splash of the reserved cooking water to ensure the sauce coats the pasta.

Step 3 Arrange in bowls and top with a few rocket leaves and grated Parmesan cheese, if desired.

Chapter Nine

FIGS, FENNEL, GORGONZOLA, & HAZELNUTS ON RYE PIZZA

Prep time: 1 hour; cooking time: 45 minutes; rising time: 2-3 hours; yield: 2 x 30cm pizzas • 5g active dried yeast • 250g strong white flour • 125g '00' flour • 125g rye flour • 12 tsp sugar • 1 tsp olive oil • semolina flour, for dusting

Topping

• 1 large fennel bulb (reserve any fronds) • 1/2 small lemon juice

• 1 tbsp olive oil • 2 medium onions, halved and very finely sliced • 14 tsp fennel seeds, coarsely crushed in a mortar • a little extra virgin olive oil, for drizzling • 12 small figs, halved •

12 12 tbsp balsamic vinegar • a little caster sugar, for sprinkling

DIRECTIONS

To make the dough, combine the yeast, 2 tbsp warm water, and 1 tbsp strong white flour in a small mixing bowl. Allow 20 minutes to'sponge' somewhere warm (this dissolves and activates the yeast). Make a well in the middle of the three flours in a large mixing bowl. To make a wet dough, combine the sponged yeast, 1 teaspoon salt, sugar, oil, and 290mL warm water in a mixing bowl. Knead for 10 minutes, or until satiny and elastic, then place in a clean bowl, cover with a cloth, and set aside to double in size for 2 1/2 to 3 hours.

Step 2 Cut the fennel bulb in half lengthwise and discard any tough outer leaves. Trim the bottoms of each, thinly slice with a knife or mandolin, and place in a bowl with lemon juice to prevent browning. Step 3 Heat the oil in a frying pan, then add the onions and a pinch of salt and cook for 7 minutes over medium heat. Season with pepper, add 1-2 tablespoons of water, cover, and cook on low heat for 10 minutes, or until softened. Cook for 3 minutes, stirring occasionally, with the majority of the fennel, as well as the fennel seeds and seasoning. If the mixture is still wet, uncover it and allow any liquid to bubble away.

Step 4 Preheat the oven to its highest setting an hour before cooking and place a baking sheet or pizza stone in the oven to heat. Place the dough on a lightly floured surface and knead it a little before halving and rolling each half.

Make a rough square or a circle out of the pieces. Lift the dough and stretch it with your fingertips while rotating it until each piece is 30-32cm across and as thin as possible with a slightly thicker edge.

5th Step

Place the pizza bases on two large baking sheets sprinkled with semolina. Top each base with the cooked onion and fennel mixture, then the raw fennel pieces, leaving a 3cm border on all sides.

Drizzle with a little extra virgin olive oil. Place the halved figs on top and drizzle with balsamic vinegar and sugar. Sprinkle some black pepper on top. Slide the first pizza onto the oven's preheated baking sheet with care. Bake for 8-12 minutes, or until golden and the figs have caramelized. Dot the pizza with cheese halfway through the cooking time. Scatter over the roasted hazelnuts and any saved fennel fronds. Repeat with the second pizza.

Chapter Ten

BACON & MUSHROOM RISOTTO

Prep: 10 mins - Cook: 30 mins - Serves 4 INGREDIENTS\s• 1 tbsp olive oil\s• 1 onion, chopped\s• 8 rashers streaky bacon, chopped\s• 250g chestnut mushroom, sliced\s• 300g risotto rice\s• 1l hot chicken stock\s• grated parmesan, to serve

DIRECTIONS

1st Step

Heat the oil in a deep frying pan and cook the onion and bacon for 5 mins to soften. Add the mushrooms and cook for a further 5 mins until they start to release their juices. Stir in the rice and cook until all the juices have been absorbed.

Step 2\sAdd the stock, a ladleful at a time, stirring well and waiting for most of the stock to be absorbed before adding the next ladleful – it will take about 20 mins for all the stock to be added. Once the rice is cooked, season and serve with the grated Parmesan.

Chapter Eleven

ROAST AUBERGINE PARMIGIANA

Prep: 20 mins - Cook: 1 hr and 15 mins - Provides food for 4

INGREDIENTS

• 2 tbsp extra-virgin olive oil\s• 2 garlic cloves , crushed\s• small bunch basil , stalks finely chopped\s• 2 x 400g cans cherry tomatoes\s• 1 tbsp chopped sundried or semi-dried tomato\s• 1 tsp clear honey\s• few thyme sprigs, leaves removed\s• 4 medium aubergines\s• 2 balls light mozzarella , thinly sliced\s• 25g breadcrumb\s• 25g parmesan (or vegetarian alternative), finely grated\s• crusty bread , to serve (optional) (optional)

DIRECTIONS

Heat 1 tbsp of the oil in a pan. Soften the garlic and the basil stalks for 1 min, without letting the garlic colour. Add both types of tomatoes, the honey, most of the thyme leaves and plenty of seasoning. Simmer for 5 mins – you don't want the sauce to reduce too much at this stage.

Step 2

Meanwhile, heat oven to 200C/180C fan/gas 6. Cut 6 slits down into the flesh of each aubergine crosswise, taking care not to cut all the way through. Season inside, then push a slice of the mozzarella and a basil leaf into each gap.

Step 3: Place the aubergines in a large baking dish with the tomato sauce (or use 4 individual dishes). Drizzle the rest of the oil on top. Cover with foil and scrunch the edges tightly. Bake for 50 minutes to 1 hour, or until soft.

4th Step

Remove the foil from the dish. Combine the breadcrumbs and Parmesan, then sprinkle the remaining thyme over the aubergines. Bake for 15 minutes more, uncovered, until the aubergines are very tender and the crumbs are golden and crisp. (Using a skewer, prod the largest aubergine in the center to see if it's ready.) Allow 5 minutes for the dish to rest before scattering the remaining basil leaves on top. If you want, serve with crusty bread.

Chapter Twelve

ONE-POT CHICKEN IN THE SPRING

Prep time: 10 minutes; cooking time: 55 minutes - Provides food for INGREDIENTS: 4 INGREDIENTS

• 1 tbsp olive oil • 8 skin-on, bone-in chicken thighs • 1 onion, sliced • 200g streaky bacon, chopped • 1 carrot, chopped • 2 large spring greens, shredded • 600ml chicken stock • 300g baby new potato • 2 tbsp crème fraîche • 2 tbsp basil pesto • crusty bread, to serve (optional)

DIRECTIONS

Step 1: In a large, heavy-based pan with a lid, heat the oil. Season the chicken with salt and pepper, then brown it all over. Place the chicken on a plate and cook the onion and bacon for 5 minutes, or until softened and lightly browned. Step 2 Return the chicken to the pan and stir in the remaining INGREDIENTS, except the crème fraîche and pesto, as well as a generous amount of freshly ground black pepper. Bring to a boil, then reduce to a low heat and cook for 30-40 minutes, or until the potatoes are tender and the chicken is cooked through.

Step 3 Combine the crème fraîche and pesto in a large mixing bowl. If desired, serve with crusty bread to mop up the sauce.

Chapter Thirteen

PESTO DEL KALE

Time to prepare: 10 minutes There's no need to cook this dish because it serves 10-12 people. INGREDIENTS • 85g toasted pine nuts • 85g coarsely grated parmesan (or vegetarian alternative), plus extra to serve (optional)

• 3 garlic cloves • 75 mL extra-virgin olive oil, plus extra to serve • 75 mL olive oil • 85 g kale

• to serve: spaghetti or linguine

DIRECTIONS

Step 1 In a food processor, whiz the pine nuts, Parmesan, garlic, oils, kale, and lemon juice to a paste. Season to taste with salt and pepper. To serve, stir in the hot pasta and top with additional Parmesan and olive oil, if desired. Step 2 To store, pour into a container or jar, drizzle with a little more olive oil, and store in the refrigerator for up to a week, or freeze for up to a month.

Chapter Fourteen

MERINGUE CAKE WITH LEMON

Preparation time: 2 hours - cooking time: 1 hour - servings: 8
INGREDIENTS FOR LEMON CURD: 16

• 75 g unsalted butter, softened • 225 g caster sugar

• 3 big eggs • 1 tbsp cornflour For the caramel sugar syrup • 85g caster sugar

300g unsalted butter, melted • 200g caster sugar • 75g light muscovado sugar • 300g self-raising flour

• 1 tsp baking powder • 25g cornflour

4 lemons, zest

1 lemon • 175g caster sugar For the Italian meringue: 300g caster sugar • 6 medium egg whites • 12 tsp cream of tartar

DIRECTIONS

1st Step

Make the curd first. Whisk together all of the ingredients in a saucepan. It will seem to have curdled, but don't fret; just place the pan over low heat and whisk regularly until the mixture is smooth and thick enough to coat the back of a spoon. Pour the mixture into a basin via a strainer. Allow to cool completely before wrapping with cling film. Place in the refrigerator until ready to use, ideally overnight.

2nd step

Heat the caster sugar in a saucepan over medium heat until it melts and begins to caramelize. Stir until the mixture is smooth and a deep golden color. Take the pan off the heat and gently pour in 50ml hot water. Take caution since it will steam and spit a bit. (If the sugar hardens, return it to the heat for 1-2 minutes to remelt it.) Stir well, then pour into a heatproof jug and fill up with a little additional hot water (approximately 10ml) to make a total of 100ml liquid. Allow to cool on one side alone.

3rd Step

Preheat oven to 180°C/160°C fan/gas 4 for the cake. Grease 3 x 20cm sandwich pans and line with baking paper on the bottom and sides.

Step 4 Using an electric mixer, cream together the butter and sugars in a large mixing basin until light and fluffy. 1 tbsp flour, 1 tbsp flour, 1 tbsp flour, 1 tbsp flour, 1 tbsp flour, 1 tbsp flour, 1 tbsp flour Step 5 Combine the remaining dry ingredients, the lemon zest, and 1/2 teaspoon salt, then stir into the butter and caramel sugar syrup mixture. Pour the batter into the muffin pans and smooth the tops with the back of a moist spoon. Preheat oven to 350°F and bake for 25-30 minutes, or until a skewer inserted into the center comes out clean. Allow 10 minutes for the cakes to cool in the pans before turning out onto a wire rack and peeling off the paper. Allow to cool fully before serving.

Step 6: While the cakes are baking, make the caramelized lemon slices. Discard the ends of the lemon and slice it into 5mm thick slices. Bring 350mL water and the sugar to a boil in a small non-stick pan. Add the lemon slices, bring to a boil for 10 minutes, then lower to a low heat and cook for another 20-25 minutes, or until the liquid has evaporated and the slices have caramelized. Remove the pan from the heat and place it on a nonstick surface. To cool, use a silicone mat or parchment paper.

Step 7: Putting the cake together. Place a sponge on a cake board or display plate the proper side up. Spread an equal layer of curd on top, leaving around 1cm uncovered. Gently place the next sponge on top and continue the procedure, ending with the final sponge on top, upside down.

Step 8 To prepare the Italian meringue, combine the sugar and 175mL water in a saucepan and bring to a boil over high heat. Boil until a sugar thermometer reads 115°C. In a large mixing bowl, combine the egg whites and cream of tartar (a tabletop mixer is ideal if you have one). Soft peaks should be achieved by whisking the egg whites (when lifting the whisk out, the peaks should slowly vanish back into the mixture). Whisk the egg whites at high speed until stiff peaks form, then gently drizzle in the hot syrup. After approximately 10 minutes, the meringue will begin to thicken and become glossy. Continue whisking until the mixture is barely heated. Use the meringue right away since it is simpler to deal with while it is warm.

Step 9 Apply a thin coating of meringue along the edge of the cake using a palette knife to level and square it up, then spread an equal layer approximately 3mm thick on top of it (see step-by-step for guidance). Fill a large piping bag with the remaining meringue and pipe vertical columns up the edge of the cake, level with the top.

Finally, pipe little meringue stars on the columns' tops. With the cake on a turntable, this is a lot simpler.

Step 10: Using a kitchen blowtorch, brown the meringue. Finally, cut the caramelized lemon slices in half and use them to adorn the cake's top. Refrigerate for up to 3 days.

Chapter Fifteen

ARTICHOKES, LEEK, & LEMON RAVIOLI

10 minutes to prepare, 10 minutes to cook, and 10 minutes to serve 2 INGREDIENTS • 280 g jar artichoke antipasto, drained (save the liquid) 1 tablespoon oil, coarsely chopped artichokes • 1 big leek, thinly sliced • 1 garlic clove, smashed • 3 tablespoons cream cheese • zest and juice one lemon

• 2 big handfuls rocket and grated Parmesan (or vegetarian substitute) to serve (optional)

DIRECTIONS

Step 1 In a large saucepan, heat the artichoke oil, then add the leek and garlic. Cook over medium heat for 5 minutes, or until the leek is tender. Heat through the artichokes, cream cheese, and lemon zest. Season with salt & pepper and a squeeze of lemon juice to taste.

Step 2 In the meanwhile, prepare the ravioli according to the package directions. Drain and stir with the artichokes and cream cheese in the pan. Serve with a sprinkling of rocket and a grating of Parmesan, if desired.

Chapter Sixteen

PORCHETTA WITH STUFFING

30 minutes to prepare - Cooking time: 3 hours and 5 minutes, plus at least 8 hours of chilling time, 1 hour of standing time, and 30 minutes of resting time Serves INGREDIENTS: 6 – 8

- 1 tbsp bicarbonate of soda • 12 kg bone-out pork belly

- 3 teaspoons fennel seeds • 1 teaspoon chilli flakes

- 1 tbsp extra virgin olive oil • 1 medium onion, finely chopped • 12 fennel bulb, hard core removed and discarded, rest finely chopped • 12 tsp coriander seeds, crushed • 2 garlic cloves, crushed • 250g minced pork shoulder • 1 slice sourdough bread, torn into small pieces • 25g toasted pine nuts • grated zest 1 unwaxed orange • 3 finely chopped dried apricots • 3 finely chopped sage leaves • 12 tbsp rosemary leaves, minced • 12 tbsp lemon juice • freshly grated nutmeg • 1 egg, beaten DIRECTIONS 1st Step

Using a sharp knife, score the pork belly skin in a cross pattern. Score immediately before the skin touches the fat, not the fat itself. Add the bicarbonate of soda to a large pot of water and bring to a boil. Lower the pork into the water, gently poach for 5 minutes, then take it from the water and cool to room temperature.

2nd step

Meanwhile, roast the fennel seeds and chilli flakes for 1-2 minutes in a dry frying pan over high heat, then transfer to a bowl and set aside to cool. Mix the spices with 1 tbsp fine sea salt in a spice grinder or pestle and mortar.

Step 3 When the pork is cold enough to handle, flip it skin-side down and puncture the flesh all over with a knife. Cover the meat with the seasoned salt rub and refrigerate for at least 8 hours or overnight. It's possible to prepare it up to 24 hours ahead of time.

4th Step

Make the stuffing the following day. In a non-stick frying pan, heat the olive oil and add the onion and fennel. Season to taste and simmer for 10 minutes over low heat. Cook for another 2 minutes after adding the coriander seeds and garlic, then add the mince. Cook for 8-10 minutes, until the mince is cooked through.

browned. Set aside to cool.

Step 5 Toss the mince and onion mixture with the sourdough, pine nuts, orange zest, apricots, herbs, lemon juice, and nutmeg in a large mixing dish. Season well, then fully combine with your hands. Remix in the egg.

Step 6: Place the pork belly skin-side down on a cutting board. Form the filling into a sausage form that runs the length of the belly. Wrap butcher's twine around the sides of the belly to secure the filling. Chill for at least 2 hours, ideally overnight, seam-side down in a roasting tin. You want the skin to be fully dry before roasting so that it crisps up.

Step 7 Before cooking the pork, take it out of the fridge and let it come to room temperature for at least 1 hour. Preheat the oven to 180°C/160°C fan/gas 4 and cook the pork for 2 hours, rotating the pan every 30 minutes or so. Cook for additional 20 minutes at 220C/ 200C fan/gas 7 after 2 hours.

A thermometer inserted into the center of the pork should register 77°C when it is done. Cover the skin with foil if it seems to be burning, but only after it has cracked.

Step 8 Remove the pork from the oven and set aside for 30 minutes to rest. Place the pork on a large chopping board when you're ready to cut it. Cut the meat into rounds using a sharp knife.

Chapter Seventeen

SEA BREAM IN RIDICULOUS WATER

Prep time: 10 minutes; cooking time: 30 minutes - Provides food for INGREDIENTS: 4 INGREDIENTS

• 2 entire sea bream or sea bass (approximately 450g each), gutted and cleaned • 2 garlic cloves, finely sliced • 12 tiny red chili, chopped • 400g small tomato (a combination of different-colored cherry tomatoes would be ideal) • 4 tbsp white wine

• a little handful of capers • parsley, chopped DIRECTIONS 1st Step

In a large, covered frying pan, heat half of the oil. Carefully place the fish in the hot oil and cook for 4-5 minutes, or until it starts to brown. Turn the fish over and distribute the garlic all over it. Add the chilli and spread it over the tomatoes after another minute of sizzling. Pour in the wine and let it boil for 1 minute, then add 100ml water and season with salt and pepper.

Step 2 Cover and cook for 15 minutes, or until the fish is cooked through — the eyes will become brilliant white and the flesh will feel softer.

Step 3 Remove each fish from the pan and place on a serving platter before returning the pan to the heat. Boil for 1 minute, then add the capers and parsley. You may either serve the fish and sauce separately now, or return them to the pan, ladle additional sauce over them, and bring the pan to the table. Just before serving, drizzle a little extra oil over top.

Chapter Eighteen

PASTA WITH CREAMY CHICKEN AND GREEN BEANS

ten minutes to prepare ten minutes to cook ten minutes to prepare ten minutes to cook ten minutes to cook ten minutes to cook ten minutes - Provides food for
INGREDIENTS: 4 INGREDIENTS

• 400g pasta shapes • 250g trimmed green beans • 1 tbsp olive oil • 1 bunch finely sliced spring onions • 2 big ready-roasted chicken breasts, chopped • 5 tbsp pesto • 3 tbsp double cream • handful grated parmesan to serve

DIRECTIONS

Step 1 Cook the pasta according to the package directions, adding the green beans for the last 6 minutes of cooking time. Drain the cooking water and set aside a few tablespoons.

In a big frying pan, heat olive oil in the meanwhile. Cook for 1-2 minutes, until spring onions are tender, then put aside.

Step 3 Heat the shredded chicken in the pan. Combine pesto and cream in a mixing bowl. Add the pasta and beans to the chicken mixture and toss to combine, adding a little of the boiling water if necessary. Season with salt and pepper, then top with Parmesan cheese.

Chapter Nineteen

COURGETTE, MASCARPONE, & SPRING ONIONS GNOCCHI

Preparation time: 5 minutes; cooking time: 15 minutes - Provides food for 2 INGREDIENTS • 300g fresh gnocchi • 1 tbsp olive oil • 1 big courgette, cut into thin ribbons with a peeler • 4 spring onions, chopped • zest 1 lemon • 2 heaping tbsp mascarpone • 50g parmesan (or vegetarian option), grated

DIRECTIONS

Step 1: Prepare the gnocchi according to the package directions. Drain and put aside, saving a ladle of the cooking water. Step 2 In a frying pan, heat the oil. Cook for 3 minutes, or until chilli and courgette are tender. Spring onions, zest, mascarpone, half of the Parmesan, and cooking water are added to the pan. Mix until smooth, then add the gnocchi and cook until hot. Step 3 Season with salt and pepper, divide into two ovenproof plates, and top with the remaining Parmesan. Serve with the dressed mixed leaves after grilling for 2- 3 minutes till bubbly.

Chapter Twenty

CANNELLONI WITH PANCAKE

30 minutes to prepare, 30 minutes to cook, 30 minutes to serve 4 INGREDIENTS • 420g pack free-range pork meatballs • 400g bag fresh spinach • 2 tbsp basil pesto • 250g tub ricotta • 1 egg beaten • 14 tsp powdered nutmeg • 8 pre-made pancakes • 500g carton passata • 1 garlic clove, smashed • 125g ball mozzarella, ripped

DIRECTIONS

Step 1 Preheat the grill to high and cook the meatballs on a baking pan for 12-15 minutes, or according to the package directions. Cut them in half and put them away.

Step 2 Place the spinach in a big colander over the sink and drain it. To wilt it, pour boiling water over it and drain completely. Squeeze off any extra liquid and cut finely when cool enough to handle.

Season to taste with salt and pepper after combining the spinach, pesto, ricotta, egg, and nutmeg.

3rd Step

Preheat oven to 190 degrees Fahrenheit/170 degrees Fahrenheit fan/gas 5. In the bottom of an ovenproof dish, pour the passata and toss in the garlic. Spread the spinach mixture on the pancakes in a long strip in the center. Fill each pancake with meatball chunks, then wrap it up to seal in the filling. Place the filled pancakes on top of the passata foundation and sprinkle with mozzarella. Bake for 30 minutes, or until the cheese has melted and the sauce is boiling. To serve, scatter basil leaves over the top.

Chapter Twenty-One

PANCETTA, SPINACH, AND PARMESAN CREAM ON GNOCCHI

15 minutes total - 4 servings • 500g gnocchi • 1 sliced garlic clove • 1 tbsp olive oil • 100ml double cream

• 1 tsp. nutmeg, grated

• 100g spinach • 12 lemon zest • 130g smoked pancetta cubes

• 25g grated parmesan cheese, plus extra for serving • 25g pine nuts, toasted

DIRECTIONS

1.

Cook and drain the gnocchi according to the package directions. Meanwhile, fry the garlic in 1 tsp oil in a small pan, then add the cream and a generous grating of nutmeg. Set aside for now. Step 2 In a frying pan, heat 2 tablespoons of the remaining oil and crisp the pancetta. Fry until the gnocchi begins to turn golden, adding a little more oil if it sticks. Season with salt and pepper and stir in the spinach and lemon zest.

Step 3 Combine the cream sauce and the Parmesan cheese. Drizzle the sauce over the gnocchi and sprinkle with pine nuts. Serve with a sprinkling of grated Parmesan cheese on top.

Chapter Twenty-Two

POLENTA CAKE WITH ORANGE INGREDIENTS

20 minutes to prepare - 45 minutes to cook - 8 servings
INGREDIENTS (8)

• 4 large eggs • 140g polenta • 200g plain flour • 2 tsp baking powder • 250g unsalted butter • 250g golden caster sugar

• lemon juice and zest • 100ml orange juice • 100g golden caster sugar • 2 oranges (less 100ml juice for the glaze) For the orange glaze

DIRECTIONS

1.

Preheat the oven to 160 degrees Fahrenheit/140 degrees Fahrenheit fan/gas. 3. Using baking parchment, line the bottom and sides of a 23cm round cake tin. Combine the butter and sugar in a large mixing bowl and cream together until light and fluffy. One at a time, add the eggs and thoroughly mix each one. After you've measured out 100ml for the glaze, combine all of the dry INGREDIENTS with the zest and juice.

Step 2 Pour the batter into the tin, smooth it out evenly, and bake for 45 minutes, or until a skewer inserted in the center comes out clean. Remove the baking sheet from the oven and cool on a wire rack. Step 3 Bring the juice and sugar to a boil in a medium saucepan to make the glaze. Allow to cool for 5 minutes after simmering for 5 minutes. Over the cooled cake, drizzle the orange glaze. Serve with a dollop of lemon ice cream (recipe follows).

Chapter Twenty-Three

PURPLE SPROUTING BROCCOLI AND ANCHOVY ORECCHIETTE

PURPLE SPROUTING BROCCOLI AND ANCHOVY ORECCHIETTE

10 minutes to prepare - 15 minutes to cook • THERE ARE ONLY TWO INGREDIENTS IN THIS PRODUCT.

• 200g orecchiette • 4 tablespoons olive oil • 6 anchovy fillets in oil, chopped (reserve 1 tablespoon oil) • 4 fat garlic cloves, thinly sliced • 1 red chili, thinly sliced

• 200g purple sprouting broccoli • 50g fresh breadcrumb

DIRECTIONS

1.

Follow the package directions for cooking orecchiette. In a separate frying pan, heat 3 tablespoons olive oil and 1 tablespoon anchovy oil. Add the garlic and chili and cook for 3-4 minutes, or until the garlic is golden brown. Cook for another 1-2 minutes, until the anchovies have melted into the sauce, then add the lemon juice. In a separate frying pan, combine the remaining olive oil, breadcrumbs, and lemon zest and cook until crispy.

Step 2 Add the broccoli to the pan when the pasta is about to finish cooking. Drain the pasta, reserving a cup of the cooking water, and combine with the garlic and anchovies in a frying pan. Stir in a splash of pasta water if it looks dry and cook for another 2 minutes over low heat. Season, then top with lemony crumbs and serve in pasta bowls.

Chapter Twenty-Four

BIRYANI WITH LESS FAT CHICKEN

Cooking time: 1 hour and 35 minutes (preparation time: 25 minutes) In addition to marinating - Serves 5 INGREDIENTS • 3 finely grated garlic cloves • 2 tsp finely grated ginger • 14 tsp ground cinnamon • 1 tsp turmeric

• 600g boneless, skinless chicken breast, cut into 4-5cm pieces • 2 tbsp semi-skimmed milk • good pinch saffron • 4 medium onions • 4 tbsp rapeseed oil • 12 tsp hot chili powder • 1 cinnamon stick, broken in half • 5 green cardamom pods, lightly bashed to split • 3 cloves • 1 tsp cumin seed

DIRECTIONS

1.

Combine the garlic, ginger, cinnamon, turmeric, and yogurt in a mixing bowl with a pinch of pepper and 14 teaspoon salt. Stir in the chicken pieces to coat them in the sauce. Refrigerate for 1 hour, or longer if you have time. Warm the milk until it is barely warm, then add the saffron and set it aside.

Step 2 Preheat the oven to 200 degrees Fahrenheit/180 degrees Fahrenheit fan/gas 3. 6. Half an onion lengthwise, set aside half, and thinly slice the other half. Pour 112 tbsp oil onto a baking sheet, scatter the sliced onion on top, toss to coat, and then spread out in a thin, even layer. Cook, stirring halfway through, for 40-45 minutes, or until golden.

Step 3: Thinly slice the reserved onion after the chicken has marinated. In a large sauté pan or frying pan, heat 1 tablespoon of oil. Cook until the onion is golden brown, about 4-5 minutes. Add the chicken, a spoonful at a time, and fry until it is no longer opaque before adding the next spoonful. Stir-fry for another 5 minutes after the last of the chicken has been added, until everything appears to be juicy. Scrape any stuck-on bits from the bottom of the pan, stir in the chilli powder, then cover and simmer for 15 minutes on a low heat. Remove the item and place it on the counter.

4)

While the chicken cooks, start the rice. In a large sauté pan, heat 1 tbsp oil, then drop in the eggs.

cardamom, cloves, and cumin seeds in a cinnamon stick Fry them for a few minutes until they release their aroma. Step 3: Add the rice and stir constantly for 1 minute. Bring to a boil after adding the stock. Reduce to a low heat and cover for about 8 minutes, or until the stock is completely absorbed. Remove the rice from the heat and cover for a few minutes to allow it to fluff up. Set aside the remaining 112 tsp oil, which has been stirred in with the garam masala. Remove the onions from the oven and lower the temperature to 180°C/160°C fan/gas 4 once they have finished roasting. 5.

Half the chicken and its juices should be placed in an ovenproof dish measuring 25 x 18 x 6cm, and a third of the roasted onions should be sprinkled on top. Remove the whole spices from the rice and spread half of it over the chicken and onions. Pour the spiced oil over the top. Add the remaining chicken and a third of the onions and mix well. Drizzle the saffron-infused milk over the remaining rice (step 4) and serve. Cover tightly with foil and heat in the oven for about 25 minutes to heat through the rest of the onions. Serve with mint and coriander leaves scattered on top.

CHILLI BLACK BEANS AND SPICY MEATBALLS

20 minutes to prepare - 25 minutes to cook • THERE ARE FOUR INGREDIENTS IN THIS PRODUCT.

• 1 red onion, halved and sliced • 2 garlic cloves, sliced • 1 large yellow pepper, quartered, deseeded, and diced • 1 tsp ground cumin • 2-3 tsp chipotle chilli paste • 300ml reduced-salt chicken stock • 400g can cherry tomatoes • 400g can black beans or red kidney beans, drained

2 spring onions, finely chopped • 1 tsp ground cumin • 1 tsp coriander • small bunch coriander, chopped, stalks and leaves kept separate • 1 tsp rapeseed oil DIRECTIONS 1.

The meatballs should be made first. Combine the mince, oats, spring onions, spices, and coriander stalks in a mixing bowl and lightly knead the INGREDIENTS until well combined. Make 12 ping-pong-size balls out of the dough. In a nonstick frying pan, heat the oil, then add the meatballs and cook until golden, turning frequently. Take the pan out of the oven.

Step 2 Add the onion, garlic, and pepper to the pan and stir-fry until the onions and garlic are softened. Pour in the stock after adding the cumin and chilli paste. Return the meatballs to the pan and cook for another 10 minutes, covered, on a low heat. Cook, covered, for a few more minutes after adding the tomatoes and beans. Toss the avocado chunks in lime juice and serve the meatballs with avocado and coriander leaves on top.

Chapter Twenty-Five

SHEPHERD'S PIE, SLOW COOKER

1 hr preparation - 5 hr cooking • THERE ARE FOUR INGREDIENTS IN THIS PRODUCT.

• 1 tablespoon olive oil • 1 onion, finely chopped • 3-4 thyme sprigs • 2 carrots, finely diced • 250g lean (10%) mince lamb or beef • 1 tablespoon plain flour • 1 tablespoon tomato purée • 400g can lentils or white beans • 1 teaspoon Worcestershire sauce

• 650g peeled and chunked potatoes • 250g peeled and chunked sweet potatoes • 2 tbsp halffat crème fraîche

DIRECTIONS

1.

If necessary, warm up the slow cooker. In a large skillet, heat the oil. Cook for 2-3 minutes after adding the onions and thyme sprigs. Then toss in the carrots and cook, stirring occasionally, until the vegetables begin to brown. Fry for 1-2 minutes, or until the mince is no longer pink. Cook for 1-2 minutes after stirring in the flour. Season with pepper and Worcestershire sauce, then stir in the tomato purée and lentils. If the mixture seems too dry, add a splash of water. Scrape everything into the slow cooker.

Step 2 Meanwhile cook both lots of potatoes in simmering water for 12-13 minutes or until they are cooked through. Drain well and then mash with the crème fraîche. Spoon this on top of the mince mixture and cook on Low for 5 hours - the mixture should be bubbling at the sides when it is ready. Crisp up the potato topping under the grill if you like.

Chapter Twenty-Six

CURRIED SPINACH, EGGS & CHICKPEAS

Prep: 15 mins - Cook: 35 mins • 2 INGREDIENTS • 1 tbsp rapeseed oil • 1 onion , thinly sliced • 1 garlic clove , crushed • 3cm piece ginger , peeled and grated • 1 tsp ground turmeric • 1 tsp ground coriander • 1 tsp garam masala • 1 tbsp ground cumin • 450g tomatoes , chopped • 400g can chickpeas , drained • 1 tsp sugar • 200g spinach • 2 large eggs • 3 tbsp natural yogurt • 1 red chilli , finely sliced • ½ small bunch of coriander , torn

DIRECTIONS

1.

Heat the oil in a large frying pan or flameproof casserole pot over a medium heat, and fry the onion for 10 mins until golden and sticky. Add the garlic, ginger, turmeric, ground coriander, garam masala, cumin and tomatoes, and fry for 2 mins more. Add the chickpeas, 100ml water and the sugar and bring to a simmer. Stir in the spinach, then cover and cook for 20-25 mins. Taste and adjust seasonings as necessary.

Step 2 Cook the eggs in a pan of boiling water for 7 mins, then rinse under cold running water to cool. Drain, peel and halve. Swirl the yogurt into the curry, then top with the eggs, chilli and coriander. Season.

Chapter Twenty-Seven

CABBAGE SOUP

CABBAGE SOUP

Prep: 20 mins - Cook: 50 mins - Serves 6 INGREDIENTS

• 2 tbsp olive oil • 1 large onion , finely chopped • 2 celery sticks , finely chopped • 1 large carrot , finely chopped • 70g smoked pancetta , diced (optional) • 1 large Savoy cabbage , shredded • 2 fat garlic cloves , crushed • 1 heaped tsp sweet smoked paprika • 1 tbsp finely chopped rosemary • 1 x 400g can chopped tomatoes • 1.7l hot vegetable stock • 1 x 400g can chickpeas , drained and rinsed • shaved parmesan (or vegetarian alternative), to serve (optional) • crusty bread , to serve (optional)

DIRECTIONS

1.

Heat the oil in a casserole pot over a low heat. Add the onion, celery and carrot, along with a generous pinch of salt, and fry gently for 15 mins, or until the veg begins to soften. If you're using pancetta, add it to the pan, turn up the heat and fry for a few mins more until turning golden brown. Tip in the cabbage and fry for 5 mins, then stir through the garlic, paprika and rosemary and cook for 1 min more.

Step 2 Tip the chopped tomatoes and stock into the pan. Bring to a simmer, then cook, uncovered, for 30 mins, adding the chickpeas for the final 10 mins. Season generously with salt and black pepper. Step 3 Ladle the soup into six deep bowls. Serve with the shaved parmesan and crusty bread, if you like.

Chapter Twenty-Eight

RED PEPPER, SQUASH & HARISSA SOUP

Prep: 15 minutes - Cook: 1 hour - Serves 6 INGREDIENTS\s• 1 small butternut squash (about 600-700g), peeled and cut into chunks\s• 2 red pepper , roughly chopped\s• 2 red onion , roughly chopped\s• 3 tbsp rapeseed oil\s• 3 garlic cloves in their skins\s• 1 tbsp ground coriander\s• 2 tsp ground cumin\s• 1.2l chicken or vegetable stock\s• 2 tbsp harissa paste\s• 50ml double cream DIRECTIONS 1.

Heat oven to 180C/160C fan/gas 4. Put all the produce on a wide baking pan and mix together with rapeseed oil, garlic cloves in their skins, ground coriander, ground cumin and some pepper. Roast for 45 minutes, moving the veg about in the tray after 30 mins, until tender and beginning to caramelise. Squeeze the garlic cloves out of their skins. Tip everything into a big pan. Add the chicken or vegetable stock, harissa paste and double cream. Bring to a simmer and boil for a few minutes. Blitz the soup in a blender, check the seasoning and add extra liquid if you need to.

Serve swirled with additional cream and harissa.

WARM CHERRY & BROWN SUGAR COMPOTE

5 minutes to prepare – 15 minutes to cook • THERE ARE FOUR INGREDIENTS IN THIS PRODUCT.

• 390g jar cherries in kirsch\s• 2 tbsp dark brown sugar\s• 4 huge scoops of vanilla ice cream\s• 50g amaretti biscuits

DIRECTIONS

Step 1\sTip the cherries and sugar into a small saucepan. Bring to a simmer over a medium heat, stirring, and leave to bubble for 10 minutes. Leave to cool somewhat.

Step 2\sScoop the ice cream into four dishes and pour over the heated compote. Crumble over the amaretti and serve.

Chapter Twenty-Nine

HARISSA-CRUMBED FISH WITH LENTILS & PEPPERS

Prep: 15 minutes - Cook: 15 mins • 4 INGREDIENTS\s• 2 x 200g pouches cooked puy lentils\s• 200g jar roasted red peppers , drained and broken into chunks\s• 50g black olives , from a jar, finely chopped\s• 1 lemon , zested and sliced into wedges

• 3 tbsp olive or rapeseed oil\s• 4 x 140g cod fillets (or another white fish)\s• 100g fresh breadcrumbs\s• 1 tbsp harissa\s• ½ small pack flat-leaf parsley , chopped

DIRECTIONS

1.

Heat oven to 200C/180C fan/gas 6. Mix the lentils, peppers, olives, lemon zest, 2 tbsp oil and some spice in a roasting tray. Top with the fish fillets. Mix the breadcrumbs, harissa and the remaining oil and add a few spoonfuls on top of each piece of fish. Bake for 12-15 minutes until the fish is done, the coating is crispy and the lentils are heated. Scatter with the parsley and squeeze over the lemon wedges.

Chapter Thirty

CRISPY ASIAN SALMON WITH STIR- FRIED NOODLES, PAK CHOI & SUGAR SNAP PEAS

CRISPY ASIAN SALMON WITH STIR- FRIED NOODLES, PAK CHOI & SUGAR SNAP PEAS

10 minutes to prepare - 15 minutes to cook • 2
INGREDIENTS\s• 2 x 100g salmon fillets (plus 2 extra 100g salmon fillets if cooking for Flaked salmon salad lunch - see

'goes well with')

• For the marinade\s• 2 tsp reduced salt tamari or soy sauce

• 2cm piece ginger, peeled and coarsely chopped or grated\s• 1 garlic clove, finely chopped\s• 2 tbsp lemon or lime juice

• 1 tsp sesame oil

• For the stir-fried noodles\s• 85g vermicelli rice noodle\s• 2 tsp rapeseed oil\s• 1 tsp sesame oil\s• 1 spring onion, trimmed and thinly sliced\s• 1 garlic clove, finely chopped\s• ½ red chilli, deseeded and finely chopped\s• 2cm piece ginger, peeled and finely chopped\s• 100g sugar snap pea

• 100g pak choi (or spinach)\s• 1 big red pepper, sliced\s• 1 tsp tamari or soy sauce\s• 1 tsp Thai fish sauce

• juice ½ lime\s• 1 tbsp coarsely chopped coriander

DIRECTIONS

Step 1\sMake the marinade by combining together all the ingredients. Place the salmon fillets in a small bowl and pour over the marinade, flipping the fish so that it's thoroughly covered. Cover with cling film and allow to sit for 10 minutes (or longer if you have time) (or longer if you have time).

Step 2\sMeanwhile, prepare the noodles following pack directions, then drain and set them in a dish of cold water. Step 3\sHeat a non-stick frying pan. Add the salmon fillets, skin-side down, and leave for 3 minutes. When the fish is somewhat crispy, turn over and fry for a further 3 minutes on the other side. Just before you remove the fish from the pan, add any leftover marinade and let it sizzle for 10 seconds. Place

2 of the fillets, skin-side up, with their juices on a platter and cover with foil to keep warm. Put the remaining 2 fillets on another dish if used for Flaked salmon salad (see 'goes well with'), cover with foil, let to cool, then chill. Step 4\sIn a frying pan or wok, heat the rapeseed and sesame oils over a high heat. Add the spring onion, garlic, chilli and ginger, and cook frequently for approximately 1 min. Add the sugar snap peas, pak choi and pepper, and sauté for another 1-2 minutes, then add the cooked noodles. Toss well, then add the soy sauce, fish sauce and lime juice, and stir until fully blended and the skillet is sizzling.

Step 5\sRemove from the heat and divide into 2 bowls. Top each with a salmon fillet and sprinkle over any juices. Sprinkle with coriander and serve.

Chapter Thirty-One

TURKEY MEATLOAF

TURKEY MEATLOAF

Prep: 15 minutes - Cook: 55 mins - Serves 4 INGREDIENTS\s• 1 tbsp olive oil\s• 1 big onion , roughly chopped\s• 1 garlic clove , crushed\s• 2 tbsp Worcestershire sauce

• 2 tsptomato purée , plus 1 tbsp for the beans\s• 500g turkey mince (thigh is best)\s• 1 big egg , beaten\s• 85g fresh white breadcrumbs\s• 2 tbsp barbecue sauce , plus 4 tbsp for the beans\s• 2 x 400g cans cannellini beans\s• 1-2 tbsp coarsely chopped parsley

DIRECTIONS

1.

Heat oven to 180C/160C fan/gas 4. Heat the oil in a big frying pan and sauté the onion for 8-10 minutes until softened. Add the garlic, Worcestershire sauce and 2 tsp tomato purée, and mix until incorporated. Set aside to cool.

Step 2\sPut the turkey mince, egg, breadcrumbs and cooled onion mix in a large bowl and season thoroughly. Mix everything to blend, then form into a rectangle loaf and put in a large roasting tray. Spread 2 tbsp barbecue sauce over the meatloaf and bake for 30 minutes.

Step 3\sMeanwhile, drain 1 can of beans alone, then add both cans into a big dish. Add the remaining barbecue sauce and tomato purée. Season and put away.

Step 4\sWhen the meatloaf has had its first cooking time, distribute the beans over the exterior and bake for 15 minutes longer until the meatloaf is cooked through and the beans are steaming hot. Scatter over the parsley and serve the meatloaf in pieces.

Chapter Thirty-Two

GINGER, SESAME AND CHILLI PRAWN & BROCCOLI STIR-FRY

5 minutes to prepare – 10 minutes to cook • THERE ARE ONLY TWO INGREDIENTS IN THIS PRODUCT.

• 250g broccoli , thin-stemmed if you wish, cut into even-sized florets\s• 2 balls stem ginger , roughly chopped, plus 2 tbsp syrup from the jar\s• 3 tbsp low-salt soy sauce

• 1 garlic clove , crushed\s• 1 red chilli , a little thinly sliced, the rest deseeded and roughly chopped\s• 2 tsp sesame seeds\s• ½ tbsp sesame oil\s• 200g raw king prawns\s• 100g beansprouts\s• cooked rice or noodles, to serve

DIRECTIONS

1.

Heat a pan of water till boiling. Tip in the broccoli and heat for only 1 min - it should still have a wonderful crisp. Meanwhile, combine the stem ginger and syrup, soy sauce, garlic and finely chopped chilli. Step 2\sToast the sesame seeds in a dry wok or big frying pan. When they're beautifully browned, crank up the heat and add the oil, prawns and cooked broccoli. Stir-fry for a few moments till the prawns become pink. Pour over the ginger sauce, then tip in the beansprouts. Cook for 30 seconds, or until the beansprouts are cooked sufficiently, adding a touch extra soy or ginger syrup, if you want.

Scatter with the chopped chilies and serve over rice or noodles.

Chapter Thirty-Three

PANEER JALFREZI WITH CUMIN RICE

PANEER JALFREZI WITH CUMIN RICE

Prep: 20 minutes - Cook: 30 mins • THERE ARE FOUR INGREDIENTS IN THIS PRODUCT.

• 2 tsp cold-pressed rapeseed oil\s• 1 big and 1 medium onion , large one coarsely chopped and medium one sliced into wedges

• 2 big garlic cloves , minced\s• 50g ginger , peeled and shredded\s• 2 tsp crushed coriander\s• 2 tsp cumin seeds\s• 400g can chopped tomatoes\s• 1 tbsp vegetable bouillon powder

• 135g paneer , chopped\s• 2 big peppers , seeded and chopped\s• 1 red or green chilli , deseeded and sliced\s• 25g coriander , chopped

For the rice

• 260g brown basmati rice\s• 1 tsp cumin seeds

DIRECTIONS

Step 1\sHeat 1 tsp in a large non-stick frying pan and cook the chopped onions, garlic and half the ginger for 5 mins until softened. Add the ground coriander and cumin seeds and fry for 1 min longer, then tip in the tomatoes, half a can of water and the bouillon. Blitz everything together with a stick blender until extremely smooth, then bring to a boil. Cover and cook for 15 minutes.

Step 2\sMeanwhile, cook the rice and cumin seeds in a pan of boiling water for 25 minutes, or until soft.

Step 3\sHeat the remaining oil in a non-stick skillet and cook the paneer till lightly browned. Remove from the pan and put aside. Add the peppers, onion wedges and chilli to the pan and stir-fry until the veg is cooked, but still has some bite. Mix the stir-fried veg and paneer into the sauce with the chopped coriander, then serve with the rice. If you're following our Healthy Diet Plan, take two parts of the curry and rice, then refrigerate the remainder for another day. Will keep for up to three days, covered, in the fridge. To serve on the second night, warm the remaining parts in the microwave until sizzling hot.

LOW 'N' SLOW RIB STEAK WITH CUBAN MOJO SALSA

Prep: 20 minutes - Cook: 3 hours and 20 mins • THERE ARE ONLY TWO INGREDIENTS IN THIS PRODUCT.

• 1 rib steakon the bone or côte du boeuf (approximately 800g)\s• 1 tbsp rapeseed oil\s• 1 garlic clove\s• 2 thyme sprigs\s• 25g butter , cut into tiny pieces\s• sweet potato fries\s• a prepared salad , to serve

For the mojo salsa\s• 2 limes\s• 1 small orange\s• ½ small bunch mint , finely chopped\s• small bunch coriander , finely chopped\s• 4 spring onions , finely chopped\s• 1 small garlic clove , crushed\s• 1 fat green chilli , finely chopped\s• 4 tbsp extra virgin rapeseed oil or olive oil

DIRECTIONS

1.

Leave the beef at room temperature for approximately 1 hour before you cook it. Heat oven to 60C/40C fan/gas 1 /4 if you want your steak medium rare, or 65C/45C fan/gas 1 /4 for medium. (Cooking at this low temperatures will be more precise in an electric oven than in a gas one. If using gas, place the oven on the lowest setting you have, and be mindful that the cooking time may be shorter.) Step 2\sPut the unseasoned meat in a heavy-based ovenproof frying pan. Cook in the center of the oven for 3 hours undisturbed.

Step 3\sMeanwhile, create the salsa. Zest the limes and orange into a basin. Cut each in half and set, cut-side down, in a heated pan. Cook for a few moments until the fruits are toasted, then squeeze the juice into the bowl. Add the remaining ingredients and season thoroughly.

4)

When the beef is done, it should seem dry on the surface, and dark pink in colour. If you have a meat thermometer, test the interior temperature– it should be 58-60C. Remove the pan from the oven and place over a high heat on the stove. Add the oil and fry the meat on both sides for a few moments until caramelised. Sear the fat for a few moments too. Smash the garlic clove with the heel of your palm and add this to the pan with the herbs and butter. When the butter is bubbling, ladle it over the steak and simmer for another 1-2 minutes. Transfer the beef to a heated platter, cover with foil, and let to rest for 5-10 minutes. Carve away from the bone and into slices before serving with the salsa, fries and salad.

ASPARAGUS & BROAD BEAN LASAGNE

35 minutes of prep time - 1 hour and 10 minutes of cooking time • 4 INGREDIENTS • 225ml whole milk • 320g frozen baby broad beans • 3 garlic cloves, chopped • 30g pack fresh basil, roughly chopped • 12 lemon, zested • 4 spring onions, chopped • 1 tsp vegetable bouillon powder

DIRECTIONS

1.

Preheat the oven to 180 degrees Celsius/160 degrees Celsius fan/gas 4. In a saucepan, bring the milk to a boil, then add the beans. Cook for 3 minutes to defrost, then add the garlic, basil, lemon zest, spring onions, and bouillon, and blend for a few minutes until smooth with a hand blender. Step 2 Pour half of the purée into an ovenproof dish that measures 20 x 26 cm. 3 lasagne sheets on top, followed by the remaining purée and peas, and finally the remaining lasagne sheets.

Step 3 Combine the cottage cheese, egg, and freshly grated nutmeg in a large mixing bowl. Pour the sauce over the lasagne, then add the asparagus and parmesan cheese. Preheat oven to 350°F and bake for 1 hour, or until golden brown and a knife slides easily through. Keeps for two days in the fridge.

TOAST WITH SMOKED CHICKPEAS

2 minutes to prepare - 10 minutes to cook • • 1 tsp olive oil or vegetable oil, plus a drizzle • 1 small onion or banana shallot, chopped • 2 tsp chipotle paste • 250ml passata • 400g can chickpeas, drained • 2 tsp honey • 2 tsp red wine vinegar • 2-4 slices good crusty bread DIRECTIONS 1.

In a pan, heat 12 teaspoons oil. Cook for 5-8 minutes with the onion before adding the chipotle paste, passata, chickpeas, honey, and vinegar. 5 minutes of seasoning and bubbling

2nd Action

The bread should be toasty. Fry the eggs in the remaining oil in a skillet. Drizzle a little oil on the toast before adding the chickpeas and fried eggs on top.

SALAD WITH SUGAR-SPICED ONIONS AND CHARRED AUBERGINES

30 minutes to prepare - 1 hour to cook - serves 4 as a main course and 8 as a side INGREDIENTS

• 1 large aubergine, thinly sliced into rounds • 1-2 tbsp sunflower oil • 50g desiccated coconut • 12 tsp turmeric • 2 x 400g cans brown lentils, rinsed and drained • bunch spring onions, sliced • small pack coriander, stalks finely chopped, leaves roughly chopped • 150g pack pomegranate seeds

3 onions, roughly sliced • 1 tbsp sunflower oil • 2 tsp each ground cumin and coriander • 2 tbsp light brown soft sugar for the sugar-spice onions

12 tsp turmeric • 1 tbsp onion seeds or nigella seeds • 2 tbsp mango chutney for the dressing

DIRECTIONS

Begin with the onions with sugar and spices. In a frying pan, combine the onions, oil, 1/2 teaspoon salt, and spices and cook for 15 minutes, or until very soft. Cook for another 2-3 minutes, stirring occasionally, until the onions are sticky and dark golden.

Step 2 In the meantime, heat a griddle pan over medium heat and brush both sides of the aubergine slices with oil. Griddle until charred and soft in batches, turning once.

Step 3 Place the onions on a plate to cool after they've finished cooking. Clean the pan, toss in the coconut and turmeric, and toast until golden brown and crisp around the edges. Set aside to cool on a plate. Combine all of the dressing's INGREDIENTS in a mixing bowl with a pinch of salt and pepper. 4)

Place the lentils, spring onions, coriander, pomegranate seeds, and cashew nuts on a large serving platter or bowl to serve. Add the aubergine slices and sugar-spiced onions, as well as the majority of the coconut. Drizzle the dressing over the majority of the salad and toss well with your hands.

To serve, scatter the remaining coconut on top and keep the extra dressing on hand to drizzle over.

SCONES WITH A SUGAR INGREDIENT

INGREDIENTS TIME TO PREPARE: 20 MINUTES - TIME TO COOK: 12 MINUTES INGREDIENTS TIME TO COOK: 12 MINUTES - TIME TO MAKE: 8

• 85 g diced butter • 350 g self-raising flour • 14 tsp salt • 12 tsp soda bicarbonate

• 4 tbsp caster sugar • 200ml milk, warmed to room temperature, plus a splash extra

DIRECTIONS

1.

Preheat the oven to 200 degrees Fahrenheit/180 degrees Fahrenheit fan/gas 6. 6. In a food processor, blend the butter and flour together. Put the salt, bicarbonate of soda, and sugar in a bowl and mix well. Stir in the milk quickly with a cutlery knife, being careful not to overmix.

2nd Action

Turn out onto a lightly floured surface and fold in half. Gently pat to a thickness of about 1in, then use a floured cutter to stamp out rounds. To make more stamps, pat together scraps. Sprinkle crushed sugar cubes on top after brushing with a little more milk. Bake for 10-12 minutes, until golden and risen on a baking sheet.

BOLOGNESE IS HEALTHY.

5 minutes to prepare; 20 minutes to cook; 2 generously; 4 as a snack 100g wholewheat linguine • 2 tsp rapeseed oil • 1 fennel bulb, finely chopped • 2 garlic cloves, sliced • 200g pork mince with less than 5% fat • 200g whole cherry tomatoes • 1 tbsp balsamic vinegar • 1 tsp vegetable bouillon powder • generous handful chopped basil

DIRECTIONS

Step 1 Boil a large pot of water and cook the linguine according to the package directions, about 10 minutes. In a nonstick wok or a large pan, heat the oil in the meantime. Cook, stirring occasionally, for 10 minutes, until the fennel and garlic are tender.

3rd Action

Stir in the pork, breaking it up as you go to avoid large clumps, until it changes color. Cover the pan and cook over low heat for 10 minutes, until the tomatoes burst and the pork is cooked and tender. Before serving, toss in the linguine, basil, and a generous amount of pepper.

SPAGHETTI FENNEL

15 minutes to prepare - 30 minutes to prepare • 2 INGREDIENTS • 1 tbsp olive oil, plus more for serving • 1 tsp fennel seeds • 2 small garlic cloves, 1 crushed, 1 thinly sliced • 1 lemon, zested and juiced • 1 fennel bulb, finely sliced, fronds reserved • 150g spaghetti • 12 pack flat-leaf parsley, chopped

DIRECTIONS

1.

Cook the fennel seeds in the oil until they pop in a frying pan over medium heat. After 1 minute, add the lemon zest and half of the fennel slices to the garlic and cook for another minute. Cook, stirring occasionally, for 10-12 minutes, or until the fennel is softened.

Step 2 In the meantime, boil a pot of salted water and cook the pasta for 1 minute less than the package instructions. Toss the pasta and a good splash of pasta water into the frying pan with tongs. Turn the heat up to high and toss everything together thoroughly. Season generously with salt and pepper, then toss into two serving bowls with the remaining fennel slices, parsley, and lemon juice. If desired, garnish with fennel fronds, olive oil, and parmesan shavings.

CHICKEN NOODLE SOUP FROM VIETNAMESE

INGREDIENTS INGREDIENTS INGREDIENTS INGREDIENTS INGREDIENTS INGREDIENTS INGREDIENTS INGREDIENTS INGREDIENTS

• 3 shallots, sliced • 3 garlic cloves, sliced • 1 lemongrass stalk, chopped • 2.5cm piece ginger, sliced • 3 star anise • 1 cinnamon stick • 1 tsp coriander seeds • 14 tsp Chinese five spice • 14 tsp black peppercorns • 1 tbsp fish sauce

• 3 large chicken breasts • 1.25-1.5 litres high-quality fresh chicken stock

assisting

• 450g rice noodles • 4 spring onions, thinly sliced on an angle • 1 carrot, shredded or peeled into ribbons with a vegetable peeler • 2 large handfuls (150g) mung bean sprouts • large bunch coriander, chopped • small bunch mint, leaves chopped

• 1 lime, cut into wedges (optional) • 1 kaffir lime leaf, tough central stalk removed

DIRECTIONS

Step 1 In a small frying pan, heat the oil over medium heat and cook the shallots and garlic until golden brown and caramelized.

Step 2 Combine the caramelized shallots and garlic, lemongrass, ginger, star anise, cinnamon stick, coriander seeds, Chinese five-spice, peppercorns, sugar, fish sauce, and chicken breasts in a large saucepan. Cover and cook for about 15 minutes at a very low temperature.

Step 3 In the meantime, cook the noodles according to the package directions until they are just al dente. To avoid them sticking together, rinse them in cold water. Drain and divide between serving bowls. Step 4\sStrain the soup through a sieve. Discard the spices. Shred the chicken and keep to one side.

Return soup to the pot and bring to a boil. Season to taste with more fish sauce if needed.

5.

To serve, ladle piping hot soup into bowls of noodles and chicken, and top with spring onion, carrot, bean sprouts, and herbs, plus the chilli, crispy shallots and kaffir lime leaf if using. Serve with a lime wedge to squeeze over, and more fish sauce and chilli to taste.

BROCCOLI PASTA SHELLS

Prep: 5 mins - Cook: 15 mins - Serves 4 INGREDIENTS\s• 1 head of broccoli, chopped into florets\s• 1 garlic clove, unpeeled\s• 2 tbsp olive oil\s• 250g pasta shells\s• ½ small pack parsley\s• ½ small pack basil\s• 30g toasted pine nuts\s• ½ lemon, zested and juiced\s• 30g parmesan (or vegetarian alternative), plus extra to serve

DIRECTIONS

1.

Heat the oven to 200C/180C fan/gas 6. Toss the broccoli and garlic in 1 tbsp of the olive oil on a roasting tray and roast in the oven for 10-12 mins, until softened.

Step 2\sTip the pasta shells into a pan of boiling, salted water. Cook according to packet instructions and drain. Tip the parsley, basil, pine nuts, lemon juice and parmesan into a blender. Once the broccoli is done, set aside a few of the smaller pieces. Squeeze the garlic from its skin, add to the blender along with the rest of the broccoli, pulse to a pesto and season well.

3rd Action

Toss the pasta with the pesto. Add the reserved broccoli florets, split between two bowls and top with a little extra parmesan, the lemon zest and a good grinding of black pepper, if you like.

CHILLI CHICKEN WRAPS

Prep: 10 mins - Cook: 25 mins • THERE ARE FOUR INGREDIENTS IN THIS PRODUCT.

• 2 tbsp vegetable oil\s• 6 boneless, skinless chicken thighs, cut into bite-sized pieces\s• 1 large onion, thinly sliced into half-moons\s• 2 garlic cloves, finely chopped\s• 3cm piece ginger, peeled and finely chopped\s• ½ tsp ground cumin\s• ½ tsp garam masala\s• 1 tbsptomato purée\s• 1 red chilli, thinly sliced into rings\s• juice ½ lemon

• 4 rotis, warmed\s• ½ small red onion, chopped\s• 4 tbsp mango chutney or lime pickle\s• 4 handfuls mint or coriander\s• 4 tbsp yogurt DIRECTIONS Step 1\sHeat the oil in a large frying pan over a medium heat. Add the chicken, brown on all sides, then remove. Add the onion, garlic, ginger and a pinch of salt. Cook for 5 mins or until softened.

Step 2\sIncrease the heat to high. Return the chicken to the pan with the spices, tomato purée, chilli and lemon juice. Season well and cook for 10 mins or until the chicken is tender.

Step 3\sDivide the chicken, red onion, chutney, herbs and yogurt between the four warm rotis. Roll up and serve with plenty of napkins

SQUASH & SPINACH FUSILLI WITH PECANS

Prep: 10 mins - Cook: 40 mins - Serves 2 INGREDIENTS • 160g butternut squash , diced • 3 garlic cloves , sliced • 1 tbsp chopped sage leaves • 2 tsp rapeseed oil • 1 large courgette , halved and sliced • 6 pecan halves • 115g wholemeal fusilli • 125g bag baby spinach

DIRECTIONS

1.

Preheat the oven to 200 degrees Fahrenheit/180 degrees Fahrenheit fan/gas 6. 6. Toss the butternut squash, garlic and sage in the oil, then spread out in a roasting tin and cook in the oven for 20 mins, add the courgettes and cook for a further 15 mins. Give everything a stir, then add the pecans and cook for 5 mins more until the nuts are toasted and the vegetables are tender and starting to caramelise.

2nd Action

Meanwhile, boil the pasta according to pack instructions – about 12 mins. Drain, then tip into a serving bowl and toss with the spinach so that it wilts in the heat from the pasta. Add the roasted veg and pecans, breaking up the nuts a little, and toss again really well before serving.

SALI MURGHI

Prep: 20 mins - Cook: 55 mins - Serves 6 - 8 INGREDIENTS

• 2½ tbsp ghee or vegetable oil • 8 chicken thighs • 1 cinnamon stick • 5 green cardamom pods , bashed, seeds removed • 1 tsp cumin seeds • 2 onions , finely chopped • 2 green chillies , roughly chopped • 3 garlic cloves , roughly chopped • 5cm piece ginger , roughly chopped • 1 tsp ground coriander • 1 tsp ground garam masala • 1 tsp Kashmiri chilli powder • ½ tsp turmeric • 3 medium tomatoes , around 300g, finely chopped (or blitzed) • 2 tbsp white wine vinegar • 2 tsp jaggery (or soft brown sugar) • 150g dried apricots (use the soft, ready-to-eat type)

• ½ small pack coriander , chopped • Sali (optional) • 1 large potato , peeled and sliced into matchsticks (see tip below)

• vegetable oil , for shallow frying

DIRECTIONS

1.

Melt 1 tbsp of the ghee in a pan and add the chicken, skin-side side down. Once the skin is golden and crisp (around 5 mins), remove from the pan and set aside (you may need to do this in batches). Melt the remaining ghee in the pan, add the cinnamon, cardamom and cumin seeds, and fry until fragrant– around 5 mins. Stir in the onions along with a big pinch of salt and fry for 5 mins until browning in places. Step 2 Blitz the green chilli with the garlic and ginger, add to the pan and cook for 2 more mins, then stir in the spices and cook for a few mins more, splashing in a little water to prevent the spices from sticking. Tip in the chopped tomatoes.

Step 3 Return the chicken to the pan and cover it in the curry sauce, then add the white wine vinegar and jaggery. Cover and cook for 30 minutes after adding 100ml water. Remove the cover and mix in the apricots and coriander, then continue to boil for another 10-15 minutes until the sauce has reduced.

Step 4: In the meanwhile, prepare the sali. Using kitchen paper, pat the potato matchsticks dry. Fill a small, deep saucepan halfway with vegetable oil and heat over medium-high heat until it's a few centimetres deep. Fry a few of the potato matchsticks at a time until golden and crisp, about a minute. Using a slotted spoon, remove the chicken, drain on kitchen paper, and season well. Serve the curry with rice.

The flowers were heaped on top of them other.

SPAGHETTI WITH ASPARAGUS AND LEMON AND PEAS

7 minutes to prepare - 12 minutes to cook - 8 servings 2 INGREDIENTS • 150g wholemeal spaghetti • 160g asparagus, ends clipped and sliced into lengths • 2 tbsp rapeseed oil • 2 leeks (220g), cut into lengths, then thin strips • 1 red chilli, deseeded and finely chopped • 1 garlic clove, finely grated • 160g frozen peas

DIRECTIONS

1.

Cook the spaghetti for 12 minutes, or until al dente, then add the asparagus for the final 3 minutes of cooking. Meanwhile, in a large nonstick frying pan, heat the oil and sauté the leeks and chilies for 5 minutes. Cook for a few minutes longer after adding the garlic, peas, and lemon zest and juice.

2nd Action

Drain the pasta and return it to the pan with 14 cup of the pasta water, tossing everything together until everything is thoroughly combined. Serve in shallow dishes with lemon wedges for squeezing over top, if desired.

SOUP WITH COURGETTE, LEEK, AND GOAT'S CHEESE

8 minutes to prepare - 17 minutes to cook - 8 servings THERE ARE FOUR INGREDIENTS IN THIS PRODUCT.

• 1 tbsp rapeseed oil • 400g leeks, carefully cleaned and sliced • 450g courgettes, sliced • 3 tsp vegetable bouillon powder, made up to 1 litre with boiling water • 400g spinach • 150g tub soft vegetarian goat's cheese • 15g basil, plus a few leaves to serve Rye bread with whole grains

DIRECTIONS

1.

In a big pan, heat the oil and soften the leeks for a few minutes. Cook for another 5 minutes after adding the courgettes. Pour in the stock and simmer for approximately 7 minutes, covered. Step 2 Add the spinach, cover, and simmer for 5 minutes to let it to wilt. Remove from the heat and blitz with a hand blender until completely smooth. Blitz again with the goat's cheese and basil. Step 3 If you're following our two-person Summer Healthy Diet Plan, divide the soup into two bowls or big flasks, then cool and refrigerate the rest for another day. To serve, reheat in a pan or microwave. If serving in bowls, top with more basil leaves and seeds, and serve with rye bread.

MOUSSAKA WITHOUT THE FAT

15 minutes to prepare - 40 minutes to cook • 4 INGREDIENTS • 200g frozen sliced peppers • 3 crushed garlic cloves • 200g extra-lean minced beef • 100g red lentils • 2 tsp dried oregano, plus extra for sprinkling • 500ml carton passata • 1

aubergine, sliced into 1.5cm rounds • 4 tomatoes, sliced into 1cm rounds • 2 tsp olive oil • 25g finely grated parmesan

• 1 tsp. nutmeg, grated

DIRECTIONS

1.

Cook the peppers gently for around 5 minutes in a big non-stick pan — the water from the peppers should keep them from sticking. Simmer for 1 minute longer after adding the garlic, then add the meat and cook until brown, breaking it up with a fork. Combine the lentils, half of the oregano, the passata, and a splash of water in a large mixing bowl. Cook, stirring occasionally, for 15-20 minutes, or until the lentils are cooked, adding extra water if necessary.

In the meanwhile, preheat the grill to medium heat. Brush the aubergine and tomato slices with the oil and arrange them on a non-stick baking pan. Season with the remaining oregano and a pinch of salt and pepper, then grill for 1-2 minutes each side until gently browned — you may need to do this in batches.

Step 3 Combine half of the Parmesan with the yogurt and a pinch of salt and pepper. Top the beef mixture with the sliced aubergine and tomato in four small ovenproof dishes. Sprinkle the remaining oregano, Parmesan, and nutmeg over the yogurt topping. 3–4 minutes on the grill, or until bubbling. If desired, serve with a salad.

SALAD WITH SESAME DRESSING FOR SALMON

7 minutes to prepare - 16 minutes to cook • THERE ARE ONLY TWO INGREDIENTS IN THIS PRODUCT. • 250g new potatoes, sliced • 160g trimmed French beans • 2 wild salmon fillets • 80g salad leaves • 4 small clementines, 3 sliced, 1 juiced • handful of basil, chopped • handful of coriander, chopped

2 tbsp finely chopped onion (1/4 small onion) • 2 tbsp sesame oil • 2 tbsp tamari • 12 lemon, juiced • 1 red chilli, deseeded and chopped

DIRECTIONS

1.

In a steamer basket set over a pan of boiling water, steam the potatoes and beans for 8 minutes. Place the salmon fillets on top and steam for an additional 6-8 minutes, or until the salmon easily flakes when tested with a fork.

2nd Action

Meanwhile, whisk together the dressing ingredients, including the clementine juice. Divide the salad leaves between two plates and top with the warm potatoes and beans, as well as the clementine slices, if eating right away. Place the salmon fillets on top, then scatter the herbs and drizzle with the dressing. If taking to work, prepare the potatoes, beans, and salmon the night before, then pack the salad leaves separately in a rigid airtight container. To keep the leaves from wilting, combine the salad ingredients and dress just before serving.

SALAD WITH COD, CUCUMBER, AVOCADO, AND MANGO

5 minutes to prepare - 8 minutes to cook • 2 INGREDIENTS • 2 x skinless cod fillets • 1 lime, zested and juiced • 1 small mango, peeled, stoned and chopped (or 2 peaches, stoned and chopped) • 1 small avocado, stoned, peeled and sliced • 14 cucumber, chopped • 160g cherry tomatoes, quartered • 1 red chilli, deseeded and chopped

DIRECTIONS

1.

Preheat the oven to 200 degrees Fahrenheit/180 degrees Fahrenheit fan/gas 6. 6. Pour half of the lime juice and a little of the zest over the fish in a shallow ovenproof dish, then season with black pepper. Bake for 8 minutes, or until the fish easily flakes but remains moist.

2nd Action

Meanwhile, combine the remaining ingredients in a mixing bowl, along with the remaining lime juice and zest. Spoon the soup onto plates and top with the cod, spooning any juices from the dish over the top.

BISCUITS FOR EASTER

Preparation time: 1 hour and 15 minutes INGREDIENTS - COOK TIME: 30 MINUTES INGREDIENTS

• 150g white caster sugar • 150g slightly salted butter, chopped • 1 large egg • 2 tsp vanilla extract or vanilla bean paste

When it comes to the iced option,

• 500g royal icing sugar • food coloring gels of your choice

• For a sloppy middle option

• 400g apricot jam (or lemon curd) • icing sugar for dusting

DIRECTIONS

1.

In a mixing bowl, weigh the flour and sugar. Rub in the butter with your fingertips until the mixture resembles wet sand and there are no butter lumps. Add the egg to the bowl along with the vanilla extract. To combine, mix briefly with a cutlery knife, then knead the dough together with your hands– don't overwork the dough or the biscuits will be tough. Form into a disc, wrap in plastic wrap, and chill for at least 15 minutes. Preheat the oven to 180 degrees Celsius/160 degrees Celsius fan/gas 4. Using baking parchment, line two baking sheets.

Step 2: Sprinkle flour on a work surface. Cut the dough in half and roll out one half to the thickness of a £1 coin. Stamp out as many cookies as you can with an egg-shaped cookie cutter (ours was 10cm long; you could also make a cardboard template to cut around), then transfer them to one of the baking sheets, leaving a little space between the biscuits.

Repeat with the remaining dough half. Use a small circular cutter to stamp holes in half of the biscuits if you want to make jammy biscuits (where the yolk would be). Only stamp holes in a quarter of the biscuits if you want to make both iced and jammy biscuits.

Step 3 Bake the biscuits for 12-15 minutes, or until they are pale gold. Cool for 10 minutes on the sheets before transferring to a wire rack to cool completely. Decorate as desired once it has cooled (see next steps). Keeps for up to five days in an airtight container.

Step 4 To ice the biscuits, combine the icing sugar and enough water to make a thick icing that will hold its shape without spreading when piped. Fill a piping bag with about a third of the icing and a very small round nozzle (or just snip a tiny opening at the tip). Pipe a border around the biscuits, then add patterns in the middle, such as lines, spots, and zigzags. Allow 10 minutes for drying. Divide the remaining icing into as many colors as you want, then dye them with the gels. Using a few drops of water, loosen each icing before transferring it to piping bags. Fill in the gaps on the biscuits with the colored icing. You have the option to

To get it into the corners, you'll need to use a cocktail stick. Allow to dry for a few hours after covering.

5.

Dust the biscuits with holes in the middle with a heavy coating of icing sugar to make the jammy middle biscuits. Spread the jam or curd generously over the entire biscuit, then top with the dusted biscuits.

NOODLES WITH GINGER CHICKEN AND GREEN BEANS

10 minutes to prepare - 15 minutes to cook • THERE ARE ONLY TWO INGREDIENTS IN THIS PRODUCT.

• 12 tbsp vegetable oil • 2 skinless chicken breasts, sliced • 200g green beans, trimmed and halved crosswise • thumb-sized piece of ginger, peeled and cut into matchsticks • 2 garlic cloves, sliced • 1 ball stem ginger, finely sliced, plus 1 tsp syrup from the jar • 1 tsp cornflour, mixed with 1 tbsp water • 1 tsp dark soy sauce, plus

DIRECTIONS

1.

In a wok, heat the oil over high heat and stir-fry the chicken for 5 minutes. Stir in the green beans for another 4-5 minutes, or until the green beans are just tender and the chicken is fully cooked. Step 2 Add the fresh ginger and garlic and stir-fry for 2 minutes, then add the stem ginger and syrup, cornflour mixture, soy sauce, and vinegar and stir-fry for another 2 minutes. Stir-fry for one minute before adding the noodles. Cook until the sauce coats the noodles and everything is hot. If desired, drizzle with more soy sauce before serving.

CURRY ROTIS WITH POTATO, PEA, AND EGG

5 minutes to prepare - 25 minutes to cook • THERE ARE FOUR INGREDIENTS IN THIS PRODUCT.

• 1 tablespoon oil • 2 tablespoons mild curry paste • 400 g can chopped tomatoes • 2 potatoes, cut into small chunks • 200 g peas • 3 hard-boiled eggs • pack rotis, warmed through

DIRECTIONS

In a saucepan, heat the oil and fry the curry paste for a few minutes. Bring to a simmer with the tomatoes and half a can of water. Cook for another 20 minutes, or until the potatoes are tender. Cook for 3 minutes after adding the peas.

2nd Action

Warm everything through by halving the eggs and placing them on top of the curry. Serve with rotis and a dollop of yogurt on the side.

BARA BRITH WITH SUGAR

15 minutes to prepare - 1 hour and 15 minutes to cook Plus soaking overnight - Serves INGREDIENTS: 12

• 400g/14oz luxury mixed fruit • 75g pack dried cranberries • mug hot strong black tea • 100g butter, plus extra for greasing • 2 heaped tbsp orange marmalade • 2 eggs, beaten • 450g self-raising flour - try a mix of wholemeal and white • 175g light soft brown sugar • 1 tsp each ground cinnamon and ground ginger • 4 tbsp milk

DIRECTIONS

1.

In a large mixing bowl, combine the dried fruit and cranberries, then pour the hot tea over them. Allow to soak overnight, covered in cling film.

Step 2 Preheat the oven to 180°C/fan 160°C/gas mark 4 4. Grease a 900g/2lb loaf tin and line the bottom with baking parchment. In a saucepan, melt the butter and marmalade together. Allow to cool for 5 minutes before adding the eggs. Remove any remaining tea from the fruit. Combine the flour, sugar, and spices in a large mixing bowl, then stir in the fruit, butter mixture, and milk until well combined. If necessary, add more milk to make the batter softly drop from the spoon. If necessary, add more milk. 114 hours, or until dark golden brown and a skewer inserted in the center comes out clean. If it begins to overcook before the middle is done, cover loosely with foil. Allow to cool completely in the tin before cutting and serving.

NOODLES WITH THAI PRAWN AND GINGER

Prep time: 15 minutes - Cook time: 15 minutes plus soaking time - Servings: 4 • 100g folded rice noodles (sen lek) • zest and juice • 112-2 tbsp red curry paste • 1-2 tsp fish sauce 1 small orange

• 85g sugar snap peas, halved lengthwise • 140g beansprouts • 175g pack raw king prawns • 2 tsp light brown soft sugar • 1 tbsp sunflower oil • 25g ginger, scraped and shredded • 2 large garlic cloves, sliced • 1 red pepper, deseeded and sliced

DIRECTIONS

Step 1: Place the noodles in a bowl and cover with boiling water. Set aside for 10 minutes to soak. To make the sauce, combine the orange juice and zest, curry paste, fish sauce, sugar, and 3 tablespoons water. Step 2 In a large wok, heat the oil and add half of the ginger and garlic. Cook for 1 minute while stirring constantly. Stir in the pepper and cook for another 3 minutes. Toss in the sugar snaps and cook for a few minutes before adding the curry sauce. Continue to cook the beansprouts and prawns until the prawns are just turning pink. Drain the noodles and combine them with the herbs and remaining ginger in the pan. Serve after mixing until the noodles are well coated in the sauce.

SOUP MAKER EASY LENTIL SOUP

5 minutes to prepare - 30 minutes to cook • • 750ml vegetable or ham stock • 75g red lentils • 3 finely chopped carrots • 1 medium leek, sliced (150g) • small handful chopped parsley, to serve

DIRECTIONS

Step 1 In a soup maker, combine the stock, lentils, carrots, and leek, and set the 'chunky soup' function. Make sure you don't exceed the maximum fill line. The soup will appear foamy at first, but don't worry; once cooked, it will disappear.

Step 2 After the cycle is finished, check to see if the lentils are tender and season generously. To serve, scatter the parsley on top.

FROSÉ PREP TIME: 5 MINUTES (plus freezing overnight) - Serves 4-6 INGREDIENTS: 1 bottle dryrosé • 300g hulled and halved strawberries • 50g caster sugar • 1 lemon juice DIRECTIONS 1.

Fill a deep roasting tin halfway with rosé and place it in the freezer overnight. Step 2 Combine the strawberries and sugar the next day and set aside for 30 minutes, or until the strawberries begin to release their juices.

To make the ultimate refreshing summer cocktail, combine the frozen rosé, strawberries, sugar, and lemon juice in a blender, then divide between glasses.

SUGAR SNAP PEAS, PAK CHOI, AND ASIAN TOFU WITH STIR-FRIED NOODLES

Preparation time: 10 minutes; cooking time: 15 minutes (plus marinating time) • THERE ARE ONLY TWO INGREDIENTS IN THIS PRODUCT.

• 2 tsp tamari or soy sauce • 195g extra-firm tofu for the marinade

• 1 garlic clove, finely chopped • 2 tbsp lemon or lime juice • 2 cm piece ginger, peeled and finely chopped or grated

• 1 tablespoon sesame oil

• 85g vermicelli rice noodle • 2 tsp rapeseed oil • 1 tsp sesame oil • 1 spring onion, thinly sliced • 1 garlic clove, finely chopped • 12 red chilli, deseeded and finely chopped • 2cm piece ginger, peeled and finely chopped • 100g sugar snap pea

• 1 large red pepper, sliced • 1 tsp tamari or soy sauce • 100g pak choi (or spinach)

• 12 lime juice • 1 tablespoon finely chopped coriander

DIRECTIONS

To make the marinade, combine all of the ingredients in a mixing bowl. Drain the tofu by placing it on a plate with several sheets of kitchen paper on top, and a heavy weight (such as a pan) on top of that. Allow at least 15 minutes. Cut the tofu into cubes and combine with the marinade in a small bowl. Cover and set aside for 30 minutes to an hour.

Step 2 In the meantime, cook the noodles according to the package directions, then drain and place in a bowl of cold water.

Step 3: Melt the butter in a nonstick frying pan. Fry the tofu pieces until they're hot and crispy. Add any remaining marinade just before removing the tofu from the pan and let it sizzle for 10 seconds. To keep the tofu warm, place it on a plate and cover it with foil.

Step 4 Heat the rapeseed and sesame oils in a frying pan or wok over high heat. Stir constantly for about 1 minute after adding the spring onion, garlic, chili, and ginger. Combine the sugar snap peas and pak choi in a large mixing bowl.

Stir in the salt and pepper for another 1-2 minutes before adding the cooked noodles. Toss well, then add the soy sauce and lime juice, mixing well until everything is well combined and the pan is hot.

5.

Remove the pan from the heat and divide the mixture between two bowls. To serve, top with tofu cubes and any remaining juices. Serve with a coriander garnish.

MUSHROOM RISOTTO IN THE SLOW COOKER

30 minutes to prepare - 1 hour to cook - 8 servings 4 INGREDIENTS • 1 onion, finely chopped • 1 tsp olive oil • 250g sliced chestnut mushrooms • 1l vegetable stock • 50g porcini • 300g wholegrain rice • small bunch parsley, finely chopped

DIRECTIONS

If required, pre-heat the slow cooker. In a frying pan, cook the onion for 10 minutes, or until tender but not browned, in the oil with a splash of water. Stir in the mushroom pieces until they soften and release juices.

Step 2 In the meanwhile, pour the stock into a saucepan with the porcini, heat to a boil, and set aside to soak. In the slow cooker, combine the onions and mushrooms, then add the rice and mix thoroughly. Pour the stock and porcini into the saucepan, leaving any sediment behind (or pour the mixture through a fine sieve). Step 3: Cook for 3 hours on high, stirring halfway during the cooking time. After that, check the consistency to see whether the rice is done. Pour in a splash of stock if it needs a bit extra liquid. Season with salt and pepper after stirring in the parsley.

Serve with a sprinkling of grated parmesan cheese on top.

CATAPLANA WITH HAKE & SEAFOOOD

15-minute prep time, 35-minute cook time

Serves THERE ARE ONLY TWO INGREDIENTS IN THIS PRODUCT.

• 2 tbsp cold-pressed rapeseed oil • 1 onion, halved and thinly sliced • 250g salad potatoes, cut into bits • 1 big red pepper, deseeded and chopped • 1 courgette (200g), thickly sliced • 2 tomatoes, chopped (150g) (optional)

• 2 tsp bouillon powder (vegetarian)

• 2 skinless hake fillets (240g pack) • 150g pack ready-cooked mussels (without shells) • 60g peeled prawns

DIRECTIONS

1.

In a large nonstick skillet with a tightly fitted cover, heat the oil. Cook for 5 minutes, or until the onions and potatoes begin to soften. Stir in the peppers, courgettes, tomatoes, and garlic, followed by the vinegar, bouillon, and 200ml water, if using. Bring to a simmer, cover, and cook for 25 minutes, or until the peppers and courgettes are very soft (if your pan doesn't have a tight-fitting lid, moisten a piece of baking paper and lay over the stew before covering to keep the juices in).

Step 2 Toss in the hake fillets, mussels, and prawns, cover, and simmer for another 5 minutes, or until the fish flakes easily when checked with a fork. Serve with a sprinkling of fresh parsley.

CAKE WITHOUT SUGAR AND LEMON DRIZZLE

10 minute prep - Cook time: 1 hour to 1 hour and 10 minutes - Cuts into eight to ten slices INGREDIENTS • 225g self-raising flour, sifted • 12 tsp baking powder • 225g xylitol (see tip below) • 2 lemons, zest only • 2 big eggs, at room temperature • 125ml sunflower oil • 1 tbsp milk

Drizzle • 1 lemon, just the juice • 50g xylitol DIRECTIONS Preheat the oven to 180°C/ 160°C fan/ Gas 4 (Step 1). Using baking paper, grease and line a 1.2 litre loaf pan (22cm x

13cm width, 7cm depth). In a large mixing bowl, combine the flour, baking powder, xylitol, and lemon zest.

Step 2 In a separate dish or jug, whisk together the eggs, sunflower oil, milk, and yoghurt, then add them into the flour mixture.

Step 3: Spoon the mixture into a pan and smooth the top. Transfer to the oven immediately and bake for 1 hour–1 hour 10 minutes on the middle shelf. If the cake is turning too dark after 50 minutes, lightly cover with foil.

Make the drizzle by heating the lemon juice and xylitol just before the conclusion of the cooking time. Stir constantly over low heat until the xylitol has completely dissolved. When the cake is done, remove it from the oven and spread the drizzle over it.

Step 5 Allow to cool completely in the tin before turning out.

CHICKEN YAKITORI

15 minutes to prepare - 25 minutes to cook - 8 servings • 100ml soy sauce • 100ml mirin • 50ml sake • 2 tbsp caster sugar • 500g boneless and skinless chicken thighs, chopped into 3cm chunks

You'll need

• 4 teppo gushi bamboo skewers, flat

DIRECTIONS

Step 1 To keep the skewers from burning, soak them in a dish of water while you prepare the rest of the meal. In a small saucepan, combine the soy, mirin, sake, and sugar and simmer over medium heat for approximately 15 minutes, or until the sauce is glossy.

Step 2 Remove the skewers from the water and thread a piece of chicken and a slice of spring onion onto each one. Repeat two more times to ensure the skewer is fully stacked. Fill all four skewers with the mixture.

Step 3 Preheat a big frying pan over medium heat; the chicken should be cooked gradually so it absorbs the sauce. Brush the skewers with the sauce after placing them in the pan. Cook for 10 minutes, turning once or twice and brushing with the remaining sauce. Serve right away.

PORK WITH HERBS AND GARLIC SERVED WITH SUMMER RATATOUILLE

15 minutes to prepare - 25 minutes to cook - 4 hours to eat (or 2 with leftovers for other meals) INGREDIENTS • 2 tsp rapeseed oil • 2 red onions, half and sliced • 2 peppers (any color), diced • 1 big aubergine, diced • 2 large courgettes, halved and sliced • 2 garlic cloves, minced — 400g can chopped tomatoes • 2 tsp vegetable bouillon • 1 thyme spig

• 475g pork tenderloin, fat trimmed, cut into 2 equal pieces • 2 garlic cloves, crushed • 1 tablespoon thyme leaves, plus a few sprigs to garnish • 1 tablespoon rapeseed oil

• to serve, brown rice or fresh potatoes

DIRECTIONS

1.

In a large nonstick skillet, heat the oil and cook the onions for 5 minutes, or until softened. Cook, stirring occasionally, for a few minutes after adding the peppers, aubergine, courgettes, and garlic. Stir in the bouillon, thyme, and basil stems after adding the tomatoes and 1 can of water. Cover and cook for 20 minutes, or until the vegetables are soft. Add the basil leaves and stir to combine.

Step 2 In the meantime, rub the pork with the garlic, then sprinkle with the thyme and black pepper, patting it in evenly. Cook the pork for about 12 minutes in a nonstick frying pan, turning frequently to brown on all sides, until tender but still moist. Cover and set aside for 5 minutes to allow flavors to meld.

Set aside half of the pork to use in the curried pork bulghar salad later in the week if you're following the Healthy Diet Plan, and keep it in the fridge after it's cooled. Refrigerate half of the ratatouille and save it for another day's ratatouille pasta salad with rocket. This step can be skipped if you're only serving four people. 4)

Slice the pork and serve with the ratatouille, brown rice or new potatoes, and more thyme on the side.

CORN SLAW AND SMASHED CHICKEN

Preparation time: 10 minutes; cooking time: 5 minutes; servings: 4 THERE ARE FOUR INGREDIENTS IN THIS PRODUCT.
• 4 skinless chicken breast fillets • 1 lime, zested and juiced • 2 tbsp bio yogurt for the chicken

• 1 teaspoon fresh thyme leaves • 14 teaspoon turmeric • 2 tablespoons finely chopped coriander • 1 garlic clove, finely grated

To make the slaw

• 1 avocado (small)

• 1 lime, zested and juiced • 2 tablespoons bio yogurt • 2 tablespoons finely chopped coriander • 160g corn, cut from 2 cobs • 1 red pepper, deseeded and chopped • 1 red onion, halved and finely sliced • 320g white cabbage, finely sliced

DIRECTIONS

Cut the chicken breasts in half, then flatten them with a rolling pin between two sheets of baking parchment. In a large mixing bowl, combine the lime zest and juice with the yogurt, thyme, turmeric, coriander, and garlic. Stir in the chicken until it is evenly coated. Allow to marinate while preparing the slaw. Step 2 Combine the avocado, lime juice and zest, 2 tablespoons yogurt, and coriander in a mixing bowl. Combine the corn, red pepper, onion, and cabbage in a mixing bowl.

Step 3 Preheat a large nonstick frying pan or griddle pan, then cook the chicken in batches for a few minutes on each side – because they're thin, they'll cook quickly. Serve the hot chicken with slaw and new potatoes on the side. If you're only cooking for two people, keep half of the chicken and slaw in the fridge for another meal (eat within two days).

MAKER OF TOMATO SOUP

5 minutes to prepare - 30 minutes to cook - 8 servings 2 INGREDIENTS • 500g ripe tomatoes, quartered or halved off the vine • 1 small onion, chopped • 12 small carrot, chopped • 12 celery stick, chopped • 1 tsp tomato purée • pinch of sugar

DIRECTIONS

Step 1: Place all of the ingredients in the soup maker and select the "smooth soup" setting. Make sure the soup maker does not exceed the maximum fill line.

Step 2 When the cycle is finished, season the soup well and taste it for sweetness. If you want more color, add a little more sugar, salt, or tomato puree.

KIDNEY BEANS & SWEET POTATO JACKETS WITH GUACAMOLE

Preparation time: 10 minutes; cooking time: 45 minutes • THERE ARE ONLY TWO INGREDIENTS IN THIS PRODUCT.

• 2 sweet potatoes • 1 large avocado • a drop of rapeseed oil

• juice 2 lime wedges plus 1 lime

• 1 red chili, deseeded and finely chopped • 2 tomatoes, finely chopped • 13 small coriander leaves, roughly chopped • 1 small red onion, finely chopped

DIRECTIONS

Step 1 Preheat the oven to 220°C/200°F fan/gas 7, oil the sweet potatoes, then place them directly on the oven shelf and roast for 45 minutes, or until pierced with a knife and tender all the way through.

Step 2 In a small mixing bowl, mash the avocado with the lime juice, then add the chilli, tomatoes, coriander, and onion.

Step 3: Halve the potatoes and top with beans and guacamole. Serve with lime wedges on the side for squeezing.

THAI CHICKEN PARCEL WITH RICE AND SUGAR SNAP PEAS

Preparation time: 10 minutes; cooking time: 20 minutes • 2
INGREDIENTS • 2 chicken breasts, skinless

• 1 pak choi, quartered • 175g sugar snap peas • small pack coriander, chopped

• 1 tablespoon fish sauce • 1 tablespoon soy sauce • 2 tablespoons rice vinegar • 2 tablespoons sweet chili sauce

• lemon juice and zest • 100g basmati rice • 1 lime • 1 tbsp Thai green curry paste DIRECTIONS 1.

Preheat oven to 220 degrees Celsius/200 degrees Celsius fan/gas 7. Cook the chicken breasts for 4-5 minutes on each side in a nonstick frying pan over high heat until browned.

Step 2 Arrange half of the coriander, pak choi, and sugar snap peas on a large piece of baking parchment on a baking tray, then top with the chicken breasts. Pour over the chicken and vegetables the fish and soy sauce, rice vinegar, sweet chilli, lime zest and juice, and curry paste, then cover with another piece of parchment. Cook for 12-15 minutes after folding up each edge to form a parcel.

Step 3: In the meanwhile, cook the rice according to the package directions. Remove the parcel from the oven and set it aside for 1-2 minutes before cutting it open and adding the remaining coriander. Serve alongside rice.

RISOTTO WITH LEEK, TOMATO, AND BARLEY AND PAN-COOKED COD

Preparation time: 10 minutes; cooking time: 20 minutes • 2
INGREDIENTS • 2 tsp rapeseed oil • 1 large leek (315g), thinly
sliced • 2 garlic cloves, chopped • 400g can barley (don't
drain) • 2 tsp vegetable bouillon • 1 tsp finely chopped sage •
1 tbsp thyme leaves, plus a few extra to serve • 160g cherry
tomatoes • 50g finely grated parmesan

DIRECTIONS

1.

In a nonstick pan, heat 1 tsp oil and fry the leek and garlic for
5-10 minutes, stirring frequently until softened. If necessary,
add a splash of water to help it cook.

Step 2 Pour in the liquid from the barley, then add the
bouillon, sage, and thyme. Simmer for 3-4 minutes, stirring
frequently. Cook for another 4-5 minutes, or until the
tomatoes soften and split, adding a drop of water if
necessary. Add the parmesan cheese and mix well.

Step 3 Meanwhile, in a nonstick pan, heat the remaining oil
and fry the cod, skin-side down, for 4-5 minutes. Cook the

fillets on the other side for a few minutes. Divide the risotto between two bowls. Serve the cod with a few thyme leaves on top, if desired.

SUPER-BREAKFAST SHAKE

Preparation time: 5 minutes (no cooking required) - Servings: 4 • 100 mL full-fat milk • 2 tbsp natural yogurt

• One banana

• 150g frozen forest fruits • 50g blueberries • 1 tablespoon chia seeds • 12 teaspoon cinnamon • 1 tablespoon goji berries • 1 tablespoon mixed seeds • 1 teaspoon honey (ideally Manuka)

DIRECTIONS

1.

Blend the ingredients until smooth in a blender. Pour into a glass and take a sip.

TORTELLINI AND GREEN MINESTRONE

5 minutes to prepare – 25 minutes to cook • THERE ARE FOUR INGREDIENTS IN THIS PRODUCT.

• 2 tbsp olive or rapeseed oil • 1 onion, chopped • 1 small leek, chopped • 1 celery stick, chopped • 3 garlic cloves, crushed • 2 bay leaves • 1 liter good-quality chicken or vegetable stock • 100g shredded spring vegetables or cabbage • 50g frozen peas • 1 lemon, zested DIRECTIONS 1.

In a large pan, heat the olive or rapeseed oil. Combine the onion, leek, and celery stick in a large mixing bowl. Cook for 8-10 minutes, or until the vegetables are softened, then add the garlic and bay leaves. Cover and cook for 10 minutes after adding the chicken or vegetable stock. Combine the spring vegetables, cabbage, peas, lemon zest, and tortellini in a large mixing bowl (spinach tortellini works well). Cover and cook for 3 more minutes, then season to taste and ladle into bowls.

CRUSHED POTATOES IN BAKED PIRI-PIRI TILAPIA

Preparation time: 10 minutes; cooking time: 25 minutes • 4 INGREDIENTS • 600g small new potatoes • 2 chunky red peppers • 1 tbsp red wine vinegar • drizzle of extra virgin olive oil • 4 large tilapia or cod pieces

• a green salad for serving

In order to make the piri-piri sauce, combine all of the ingredients in a mixing bowl.

• 6 hot pickled peppers (I used Peppadew) • 1 teaspoon chili flakes • 2 garlic cloves • 1 lemon juice and zest

• 1 tbsp smoked paprika • 2 tbsp extra virgin olive oil • 1 tbsp red wine vinegar

DIRECTIONS

1.

Preheat oven to 220°C/200°C fan/gas mark 7. 7. Drain the potatoes after they've been cooked until they're knife-tender. Using the back of a spatula, gently crush the cookies on a large baking tray. Roast for 25 minutes after adding the peppers, drizzling with vinegar and oil, seasoning well.

Step 2 Put the piri-piri ingredients in a food processor with some salt. Purée until fine, then pour into a bowl. Put the fish on a baking tray and spoon over some of the piri-piri sauce. Season and bake for the final 10 mins of the potatoes' cooking time. Serve everything with the extra sauce and a green salad on the side.

ALL-IN–ONE CHICKEN WITH WILTED SPINACH

Prep: 20 mins - Cook: 1 hr - Serves THERE ARE ONLY TWO INGREDIENTS IN THIS PRODUCT.

• 2 beetroot , peeled and cut into small chunks • 300g celeriac , cut into small chunks • 2 red onions , quartered • 8 garlic cloves , 4 crushed, the rest left whole, but peeled • 1 tbsp rapeseed oil • 1½ tbsp fresh thyme leaves , plus extra to serve • 1 lemon , zested and juiced • 1 tsp fennel seeds • 1 tsp English mustard powder • 1 tsp smoked paprika • 4 tbsp bio yogurt • 4 bone-in chicken thighs , skin removed • 260g bag spinach DIRECTIONS 1.

Preheat the oven to 200 degrees Fahrenheit/180 degrees Fahrenheit fan/gas 6. 6. Tip the beetroot, celeriac, onions and whole garlic cloves into a shallow roasting tin. Add the oil, 1 tbsp thyme, half the lemon zest, fennel seeds and a squeeze of lemon juice, then toss together. Roast for 20 mins while you prepare the chicken. Step 2 Stir the mustard powder and paprika into 2 tbsp yogurt in a bowl. Add half the crushed garlic, the remaining lemon zest and thyme, and juice from half the lemon. Add the chicken and toss well until it's coated all over. Put the chicken in the tin with the veg and roast for 40 mins until the chicken is cooked through and the vegetables are tender.

Step 3 About 5 mins before the chicken is ready, wash and drain the spinach and put it in a pan with the remaining crushed garlic. Cook until wilted, then turn off the heat and stir in the remaining yogurt. Scatter some extra thyme over the chicken and vegetables, then serve.

APPLE & ALMOND CAKE

Prep: 10 mins - Cook: 35 mins - 40 mins • 8 INGREDIENTS

• 125ml(½ cup) olive oil • 140g(½ cup) maple syrup or agave syrup • 2 eggs

• 130g (1/2 cup) apple sauce (shop-bought or homemade) • 185g (2 cups) ground almonds • 1 tsp baking powder • 1 tsp cinnamon

For the topping • 1 apple , skin-on, cored and diced • tiny splash olive oil • 1 tbsp maple syrup • ½ tsp cinnamon DIRECTIONS 1.

Heat oven to 190C/170C fan/gas 5, and lightly oil a 20cm springform tin and line the base with a circle of baking parchment.

Step 2 In a stand mixer, or using a hand blender, whizz together the oil and maple syrup for 30 secs. Add the eggs and whizz for another 1 min before adding the apple sauce and blending for a further 30 secs. Tip in the ground almonds, baking powder, 1 tsp salt and cinnamon, blend for 30 secs and your batter is done. Pour it into the tin, and bake for around 30-40 mins or until the top is a deep golden brown, the cake is coming away from the sides a little, and a skewer inserted into the centre comes out clean.

Step 3 While it's cooking, make the topping. In a small frying pan, cook the apple gently with the rest of the topping INGREDIENTSand ½ tsp salt until the apple is soft and gently caramelised. When the cake is ready, scatter the bronzed apple chunks on top of the cake. You could also make it with chunks of caramelised peach or plum on top, or some cherry compote, or any berries which you have softened in a pan with a little water and maple syrup. Eat warm, as a pudding, with a spoonful of Greek yogurt, or cold with a cup of tea or coffee.

EASY VEGAN PHO

Prep: 10 mins - Cook: 20 mins - Serves 2 INGREDIENTS • 100g rice noodles • 1 tsp Marmite • 1 tsp vegetable oil • 50g chestnut mushrooms , sliced • 1 leek , sliced • 2 tbsp soy sauce

assisting

• 1 red chilli , sliced (deseeded if you don't like it too hot) • ½ bunch mint , leaves picked and stalk discarded • handful salted peanuts

• sriracha , to serve DIRECTIONS Step 1 Tip the noodles into a bowl and cover with boiling water. Leave to stand for 10 mins, then drain, rinse in cold water and set aside.

Step 2 In a jug, mix the Marmite with 500ml boiling water. Set aside while you cook the vegetables.

Step 3 Heat the oil in a saucepan, then add the mushrooms and leek. Cook for 10-15 mins until softened and beginning to colour, then add the soy sauce and Marmite and water mixture and stir. Bring to the boil for 5 mins.

Step 4 Divide the noodles between two deep bowls, then ladle over the hot broth. Top with the chilli slices, mint leaves and peanuts, and serve with some sriracha on the side.

SEARED BEEF SALAD WITH CAPERS & MINT

Prep: 10 mins - Cook: 12 mins - Serves 2 INGREDIENTS • 150g new potatoes , thickly sliced • 160g fine green beans , trimmed and halved • 160g frozen peas • rapeseed oil , for brushing • 200g lean fillet steak , trimmed of any fat • 160g romaine lettuce , roughly torn into pieces

For the dressing • 1 tbsp extra virgin olive oil • 2 tsp cider vinegar • ½ tsp English mustard powder • 2 tbsp chopped mint • 3 tbsp chopped basil • 1 garlic clove , finely grated • 1 tbsp capers DIRECTIONS Step 1 Cook the potatoes in a pan of simmering water for 5 mins. Add the beans and cook 5 mins more, then tip in the peas and cook for 2 mins until all the vegetables are just tender. Drain.

Step 2 Meanwhile, measure all the dressing ingredients in a large bowl and season with black pepper. Stir and crush the herbs and capers with the back of a spoon to intensify their flavours.

Step 3 Brush a little oil over the steak and grind over some black pepper. Heat a non-stick frying pan over a high heat and cook the steak for 4 mins on one side and 2-3 mins on the other, depending on the thickness and how rare you like it. Transfer to a plate to rest while you carry on with the rest of the salad. Step 4 Mix the warm vegetables into the dressing until well coated, then add the lettuce and toss again. Pile onto plates. Slice the steak and turn in any dressing left in the bowl, add to the salad and serve while still warm.

MINTY GRIDDLED CHICKEN & PEACH SALAD

10 minutes to prepare - 15 minutes to cook • THERE ARE ONLY TWO INGREDIENTS IN THIS PRODUCT.

• 1 lime , zested and juiced • 1 tbsp rapeseed oil • 2 tbsp mint , finely chopped, plus a few leaves to serve • 1 garlic clove , finely grated • 2 skinless chicken breast fillets (300g) • 160g fine beans , trimmed and halved • 2 peaches (200g), each cut into 8 thick wedges

• 1 red onion , cut into wedges

• 1 large Little Gem lettuce (165g), roughly shredded • ½ x 60g pack rocket • 1 small avocado , stoned and sliced • 240g cooked new potatoes

DIRECTIONS

Step 1 Mix the lime zest and juice, oil and mint, then put half in a bowl with the garlic. Thickly slice the chicken at a slight angle, add to the garlic mixture and toss together with plenty of black pepper. Step 2 Cook the beans in a pan of water for 3-4 mins until just tender. Meanwhile, griddle the chicken and onion for a few mins each side until cooked and tender. Transfer to a plate, then quickly griddle the peaches. If you don't have a griddle pan, use a non-stick frying pan with a drop of oil. Step 3 Toss the warm beans and onion in the remaining mint mixture, and pile onto a platter or into individual shallow bowls with the lettuce and rocket. Top with the avocado, peaches and chicken and scatter over the mint. Serve with the potatoes while still warm.

PARMA PORK WITH POTATO SALAD

Prep: 15 minutes - Cook: 15 mins • THERE ARE ONLY TWO INGREDIENTS IN THIS PRODUCT.

• 175g new potatoes (we used Jersey Royals), scrubbed and thickly sliced • 3 celery sticks, thickly sliced • 3 tbsp bio yogurt • 2 gherkins (about 85g each), sliced • ¼ tsp caraway seeds • ½ tsp Dijon mustard • 2 x 100g pieces lean pork tenderloin • 2 tsp chopped sage • 2 slices Parma ham • 1 tsp rapeseed oil • 2 tsp balsamic vinegar • 2 handfuls salad leaves

DIRECTIONS

1.

Bring a pan of water to the boil, add the potatoes and celery and cook for 8 mins. Meanwhile, mix the yogurt, guerkins, caraway and mustard in a bowl. When the potatoes and celery are cooked, drain and set aside for a few mins to cool a little.

Step 2 Bash the pork pieces with a rolling pin to flatten them. Sprinkle over the sage and some pepper, then top each with a slice of Parma ham. Heat the oil in a non-stick pan, add the pork and cook for a couple of mins each side, turning carefully. Add the balsamic vinegar and let it sizzle in the pan.

Step 3 Stir the potatoes and celery into the dressing and serve with the pork, with some salad leaves on the side.

YAKI UDON

Prep: 10 mins - Cook: 5 mins • 2 INGREDIENTS • 250g dried udon noodles (400g frozen or fresh) • 2 tbsp sesame oil

• 1 onion, thickly sliced • ¼ head white cabbage, roughly sliced • 10 shiitake mushrooms • 4 spring onions, finely sliced

For the sauce • 4 tbsp mirin • 2 tbsp soy sauce • 1 tbsp caster sugar • 1 tbsp Worcestershire sauce (or vegetarian alternative)

DIRECTIONS

1.

Boil some water in a large saucepan. Add 250ml cold water and the udon noodles. (As they are so thick, adding cold water helps them to cook a little bit slower so the middle cooks through). If using frozen or fresh noodles, cook for 2 mins or until al dente; dried will take longer, about 5-6 mins. Drain and leave in the colander.

2nd Action

Heat 1 tbsp of the oil, add the onion and cabbage and sauté for 5 mins until softened. Add the mushrooms and some spring onions, and sauté for 1 more min. Pour in the remaining sesame oil and the noodles. If using cold noodles, let them heat through before adding the INGREDIENTS for the sauce– otherwise tip in straight away and keep stir-frying until sticky and piping hot.

Sprinkle with the remaining spring onions.

MUSHROOM & POTATO SOUP

Prep: 15 mins - Cook: 30 mins - Serves 4 INGREDIENTS • 1 tbsp rapeseed oil • 2 large onions , halved and thinly sliced • 20g dried porcini mushrooms • 3 tsp vegetable bouillon powder

• 300g chestnut mushrooms , chopped • 3 garlic cloves , finely grated • 300g potato , finely diced • 2 tsp fresh thyme • 4 carrots , finely diced • 2 tbsp chopped parsley • 8 tbsp bio yogurt • 55g walnut pieces DIRECTIONS Step 1 Heat the oil in a large pan. Tip in the onions and fry for 10 mins until golden. Meanwhile, pour 1.2 litres boiling water over the dried mushrooms and stir in the bouillon.

Step 2 Add the fresh mushrooms and garlic to the pan with the potatoes, thyme and carrots, and continue to fry until the mushrooms soften and start to brown.

Step 3 Pour in the dried mushrooms and stock, cover the pan and leave to simmer for 20 mins. Stir in the parsley and plenty of pepper. Ladle into bowls and serve each portion topped with 2 tbsp yogurt and a quarter of the walnuts. The rest can be chilled and reheated the next day.

COCONUT CRÊPES WITH RASPBERRY SAUCE

Prep: 10 mins - Cook: 25 mins - Serves 6 INGREDIENTS

For the raspberry sauce

• 200g raspberries • 2 tsp cornflour • 2 tsp maple syrup

For the coconut crêpes • 140g plain flour • 2 large eggs • 300ml coconut milk • 2 tbsp toasted desiccated coconut • a little sunflower oil , for frying

DIRECTIONS

1.

Set aside 6 of the raspberries. Mix the cornflour with 1 tbsp water until smooth. Measure 300ml water in a pan, and stir in the cornflour paste. Heat, stirring, until thickened. Add the remaining raspberries and cook gently, mashing the berries to a pulp. Strain the mixture through a sieve into a bowl to remove the seeds, pushing through as much of the mixture as you can. Quarter the reserved raspberries and add to the sauce, along with the maple syrup.

Step 2 To make the crêpes, tip the flour and a pinch of salt into a large jug, then beat in the eggs, coconut milk, 200ml water and 11/2 tbsp toasted coconut to make a batter the consistency of double cream. Thin with a little more water if it is too thick. Heat a small frying pan with a dash of oil, then pour in a little batter, swirling the pan so that it completely covers the base. Leave to set over the heat for 1 min, then carefully flip it over and cook the other side for a few secs more. Transfer to a plate and repeat with the remaining batter until you haveat least 12. Stir the batter to redistribute the coconut as you use it. Serve 2 crêpes per person with a drizzle of the sauce and a little of the remaining toasted coconut.

LOW-FAT CHERRY CHEESECAKE

Prep: 1 hr - Cook: 30 mins Plus overnight chilling - Cuts into 8 slices INGREDIENTS • 25g butter , melted • 140g amaretti biscuit , crushed • 3 sheets leaf gelatine • zest and juice 1 orange

• 2 x 250g tubs quark • 250g tub ricotta • 2 tsp vanilla extract • 100g icing sugar • For the topping • 400g fresh cherry , stoned • 5 tbsp cherry jam • 1 tbsp cornflour DIRECTIONS Step 1 Line the sides of a 20cm round loose-bottomed cake tin with baking parchment. Stir the butter into twothirds of the biscuit crumbs, and reserve the rest. Sprinkle the buttery crumbs over the base of the tin and press down. Soak the gelatine in cold water for 5-10 mins until soft.

Step 2 Warm the orange juice in a small pan or the microwave until almost boiling. Squeeze the gelatine of excess water, then stir into the juice to dissolve.

Step 3 Beat the quark, ricotta, vanilla and icing sugar together with an electric whisk until really smooth. Then, with the beaters still running, pour in the juice mixture and beat to combine. Pour the cheesecake mixture over the crumbs and smooth the top. Cover with cling film and chill overnight.

Step 4 To make the topping, put the cherries in a pan with the orange zest and 100ml water. Cook, covered, for 15 mins until the cherries are softened. Put one-third of the cherries in a bowl and mash with a potato masher to give you a chunky compote. Return to the pan, add the jam, cornflour and 2 tbsp water, and mix to combine. Cook until thickened and saucy – if the sauce is too dry, add a splash more water. Cool to room temperature. 5.

Just before serving, carefully remove the cheesecake from the tin and peel off the parchment. Scatter over the remaining biscuit crumbs and some cherry sauce. Serve in slices with the remaining cherry sauce alongside.

JAM TURNOVERS

Prep: 10 mins - Cook: 20 mins - Serves 6 INGREDIENTS • 320g sheet puff pastry • 1 heaped tbsp jam (apricot, raspberry or strawberry work well) • 1 beaten egg

• icing sugar , for dusting • clotted cream , to serve

DIRECTIONS

1.

Heat the oven to 200C/180C fan/gas 6. Unravel the puff pastry on a lightly floured surface. Cut the pastry into six squares. Spoon the jam in the centre of each pastry square. Seal the edges by pressing down with a fork and brush with the egg. Lay on a lined baking sheet and bake for 20 mins. Dust with the icing sugar and serve with the clotted cream.

VEGGIE OKONOMIYAKI

Prep: 15 mins - Cook: 10 mins • 2 INGREDIENTS • 3 large eggs • 50g plain flour • 50ml milk • 4 spring onions , trimmed and sliced • 1 pak choi , sliced • 200g Savoy cabbage , shredded • 1 red chilli , deseeded and finely chopped, plus extra to serve • ½ tbsp low-salt soy sauce • ½ tbsp rapeseed oil • 1 heaped tbsp low-fat mayonnaise • ½ lime , juiced • sushi ginger , to serve (optional) • wasabi , to serve (optional)

DIRECTIONS

1.

Whisk together the eggs, flour and milk until smooth. Add half the spring onions, the pak choi, cabbage, chilli and soy sauce. Heat the oil in a small frying pan and pour in the batter. Cook, covered, over a medium heat for 7-8 mins. Flip the okonomiyaki into a second frying pan, then return it to the heat and cook for a further 7-8 mins until a skewer inserted into it comes out clean.

Step 2 Mix the mayonnaise and lime juice together in a small bowl. Transfer the okonomiyaki to a plate, then drizzle over the lime mayo and top with the extra chilli and spring onion and the sushi ginger, if using. Serve with the wasabi on the side, if you like.

CHICKEN STEW WITHOUT THE WORK

Preparation time: 10 minutes; cooking time: 50 minutes; servings: 6 INGREDIENTS: 4 INGREDIENTS

• 1 tablespoon olive oil • 1 bunch spring onions, sliced, white and green parts separated • 1 small swede (350g), peeled and chopped into small pieces • 400g potatoes, peeled and chopped into small pieces • 8 skinless boneless chicken thighs • 1 tablespoon Dijon mustard • 500ml chicken stock • 200g Savoy cabbage or spring cabbage, sliced • 2 teaspoon cornflour (optional) (optional)

DIRECTIONS

1st Step

In a large saucepan, warm the oil. To soften the white spring onion slices, add them to the pan and cook for 1 minute. Cook for another 2-3 minutes after adding the swede and potatoes, then add the chicken, mustard, and stock. Cook for 35 minutes, or until the vegetables are tender and the chicken is fully cooked.

Step 2 Cook for another 5 minutes after adding the cabbage. If the stew appears to be too thin, combine the cornflour with 1 tablespoon cold water and pour a couple of teaspoons into the pan; allow the stew to bubble and thicken before checking. If the stew is still too thin, add a little more cornflour mixture and let it bubble and thicken a little more. Step 3 Season to taste with salt and pepper, then ladle the stew into deep bowls. Serve with crusty bread or warm cheese scones, if desired.

CAKE FOR A LAST-MINUTE CHRISTMAS LOAF

Prep time: 25 minutes; cooking time: 1 hour and 15 minutes
2 hr soak time - Serves INGREDIENTS: TEN

• 200g raisins and sultanas • 50g sour cherries • 100g dried figs, chopped • 150g mixed peel • 1 orange, zested and juiced • 250ml brandy • 115g butter, plus extra melted for the tin • 115g muscovado sugar • 4 eggs, beaten (optional)

DIRECTIONS

1st Step

Combine the fruit and peel with the orange juice and zest, as well as 150ml of brandy, in a mixing bowl. Stir well, then place in a warm place for 2 hours to plump up the fruit.

2nd step

Preheat the oven to 170°C/150°C fan/gas 3. 4. Line a 900g loaf tin with baking parchment after brushing it with melted butter. Mix the muscovado sugar and butter until light and fluffy, then add the eggs one at a time, beating well after each addition. Except for the remaining brandy and icing sugar, combine the fruit and the remaining ingredients in a mixing bowl. Spoon the batter into the loaf tin, set it in a deep tray, and bake for 1 hour 15 minutes to 1 hour 30 minutes, or until a skewer inserted into the center comes out clean. Remove the pan from the oven and immediately pour the brandy on top (this makes it easier for the cake to soak it up). Allow to cool completely before dusting with icing sugar, if desired.

PRAWNS AND GREEN CHOWDER

Prep time: 10 minutes; cooking time: 20 to 30 minutes - Provides food for INGREDIENTS: 4 INGREDIENTS

• 1 tbsp olive oil • 1 onion, finely chopped • 1 celery stick, finely chopped • 1 garlic clove • 300g petit pois • 200g pack sliced kale • 2 potatoes, finely chopped

DIRECTIONS

1st Step

In a medium saucepan, heat the oil. Cook for 5-6 minutes, until the onion and celery are softened but not coloured. Cook for an additional minute after adding the garlic. After that, add the petit pois, kale, and potatoes, along with the stock cube and 750ml water. Bring to a boil, then reduce to a low heat and cook for 10-12 minutes, or until the potatoes are soft.

Step 2 Whizz 34% of the mixture in a food processor until smooth. If it's too thick, thin it out with a little more water or stock. Return half of the prawns to the pan with the mixture.

Step 3 Divide among four bowls and top with the remaining prawns. It's possible to freeze it for up to a month. Once the prawns have defrosted, add them to the pan.

BRUNCH OF MUSHROOMS

Preparation time: 5 minutes; cooking time: 12 to 15 minutes - Provides food for 250g mushrooms • 1 garlic clove • 1 tbsp olive oil • 160g bag kale • 4 eggs DIRECTIONS 1st Step

Cut the mushrooms into slices and crush the garlic clove. In a large nonstick frying pan, heat the olive oil, then fry the garlic for 1 minute over low heat. Cook the mushrooms until they are soft. After that, add the kale. If the kale won't fit all of it in the pan, start with half and stir until wilted, then finish with the rest. Season when all of the kale has wilted. Step 2: Crack the eggs into the pan and cook them gently for 2-3 minutes. Cover for another 2-3 minutes, or until the eggs are cooked to your liking. Serve with crusty bread.

CAIPIROSKA

5 minute prep time - 4 servings 1 INGREDIENTS: 1 lime, 2 teaspoons golden granulated sugar, 50 mL vodka, crushed ice DIRECTIONS 1st Step

Cut the lime into small chunks and place them in the bottom of a sturdy tumbler, along with the golden granulated sugar. If you don't have a muddler, a pestle and mortar will suffice. Step 2 Fill the tumbler halfway with crushed ice, then pour in the vodka. Serve after thoroughly mixing all of the ingredients together.

PINEAPPLE RICE WITH THAI FRIED PRAWN

Prep time: 10 minutes; cooking time: 15 minutes - Provides food for INGREDIENTS: 4 INGREDIENTS

• 2 tbsp sunflower oil • 1 green pepper, deseeded and chopped into small chunks • 140g pineapple, chopped into bite-sized chunks • 3 tbsp Thai green curry paste • 4 tbsp light soy sauce, plus extra to serve

• 2 large beaten eggs • 300g cooked basmati rice (brown, white, or a mix - about 140g uncooked rice)

• 140g frozen peas • 225g drained can bamboo shoots • 250g frozen prawns, cooked or raw • 2-3 limes, 1 juiced, the rest cut into wedges to serve (optional)

DIRECTIONS

Step 1 In a wok or nonstick frying pan, heat the oil and fry the spring onion whites for 2 minutes, or until softened. Stir in the pepper for 1 minute, then the pineapple for another 1 minute, before adding the green curry paste and soy sauce.

Step 2 Stir in the rice until it is piping hot, then push the rice to one side of the pan while scrambling the eggs on the other. Heat the peas, bamboo shoots, and prawns with the rice and eggs for 2 minutes, or until the prawns are hot and the peas are tender. Finally, if using, add the spring onion greens, lime juice, and coriander. Serve with extra lime wedges and soy sauce in bowls.

LUNCH BOWL WITH FETA & CLEMENTINE

15 minutes to prepare, 15 minutes to cook - Provides food for 2 INGREDIENTS • 1 red onion, halved and thinly sliced • 1 lemon, zested and juiced • 2 clementines, 1 zested, flesh sliced • 2 garlic cloves, chopped • 400g can green lentils,

drained • 1 tbsp balsamic vinegar • 12 tbsp rapeseed oil • 1 red pepper, quartered and sliced • 60g feta, crumbled

DIRECTIONS

1st Step

Combine the onion, lemon juice, lemon and clementine zest, and garlic in a bowl.

Step 2 Divide the lentils between two bowls or lunchboxes and drizzle with the balsamic vinegar and 1 tablespoon of olive oil. In a large nonstick wok, heat the remaining oil, add the pepper, and stir-fry for 3 minutes. Add half of the onion and cook until it is tender. Place the clementines, remaining onions, feta, mint, and walnut pieces on top of the lentils.

SOUP WITH CARROTS AND GINGER

15 minutes to prepare - 25 to 30 minutes to cook - 4 to 6 people INGREDIENTS: 4 INGREDIENTS

• 1 tbsp rapeseed oil • 1 large chopped onion • 2 tbsp coarsely grated ginger • 2 garlic cloves, sliced • 12 tsp ground nutmeg • 850ml vegetable stock • 500g carrot (preferably organic), sliced (no need to drain)

• 4 tbsp almonds in their skins, cut into slivers • nutmeg

Step 1 Heat the oil in a large skillet, then add the onion, ginger, and garlic and cook for 5 minutes, or until softened. Cook for an additional minute after adding the nutmeg.

Step 2 Add the stock, carrots, beans, and their liquid, then cover and cook for 20-25 minutes, or until the carrots are tender.

Step 3 Scoop a third of the mixture into a bowl and blitz the rest in a food processor or with a hand blender until smooth. Return all of the ingredients to the pan and heat until they are bubbling. Serve with the almonds and nutmeg on top.

BUTTER BACON FRENCH TOAST

Preparation time: 5 minutes Cooking time: 25 minutes - Provides food for 2 INGREDIENTS • 2 eggs • 180ml milk • 1 tbsp caster sugar • 4 slices white bread • 2 tbsp butter • 4 rashers back bacon, grilled • icing sugar and date syrup to serve

DIRECTIONS

1st Step

In a mixing bowl, whisk together the eggs, milk, and sugar. In a large mixing bowl, soak the white sliced bread in the mixture.

Step 2 In a nonstick frying pan, melt 1 tablespoon butter and fry two slices of soaked bread until golden and crisp, about 3–4 minutes on each side. Remove the French toast from the pan and sandwich 2 slices of bacon between the slices. To make the other sandwich, repeat with the remaining soaked bread.

Step 3 Garnish with icing sugar and a drizzle of maple syrup.

SOUP WITH MISO MUSHROOMS AND TOFU NOODLE

Preparation time: 10 minutes; cooking time: 15 minutes; servings: 4 1 INGREDIENTS • 1 tbsp rapeseed oil • 70g sliced mixed mushrooms • 50g smoked tofu • 12 tbsp brown rice miso paste • 50g dried buckwheat or egg noodles • 2 shredded spring onions

DIRECTIONS

1st Step

In a frying pan over medium heat, heat half of the oil. Fry the mushrooms for 5-6 minutes, or until golden brown. Using a slotted spoon, transfer to a bowl and set aside. In the same pan, add the remaining oil and fry the tofu for 3-4 minutes, or until evenly golden.

Step 2 In a jug, combine the miso paste and 325ml boiling water. Cook the noodles according to the package directions, then drain and place in a bowl. Add the mushrooms and tofu, then pour the miso broth on top. Just before serving, scatter the spring onions on top.

SHELLS OF SAUSAGE AND BUTTERNUT SQUASH

15 minutes to prepare - 35 minutes to cook - 8 servings 4 INGREDIENTS • 1 medium butternut squash, peeled and cut into medium chunks • 12 tbsp olive oil • 2 crushed garlic cloves • 1 fennel bulb, thinly sliced (keep the green fronds to serve) • 4 spring onions, thinly sliced • 2 tsp chilli flakes • 1 tsp fennel seeds • 300g large pasta shells

Step 1: Toss the squash with a splash of water in a microwave-safe bowl. Cover with cling film and cook for 10 minutes on high, or until soft. Place in a blender.

Step 2 In the meantime, heat 1 tbsp olive oil in a frying pan over medium heat. Combine the garlic, sliced fennel, spring onions, half of the chilli flakes, half of the fennel seeds, and a splash of water in a large mixing bowl. Cook for 5 minutes, stirring occasionally, until softened. Squash should be scraped into the blender. Blend until smooth, adding water as needed to achieve a creamy consistency. Season to taste with salt and pepper.

Step 3 Boil a pot of water and cook the pasta for 1 minute less than the package suggests. Return the frying pan to the heat (no need to clean it first – it's all about the flavor). Pour in the remaining oil, squeeze the sausagemeat out of the skins, and season with the remaining chilli and fennel seeds. Fry until the sausagemeat is browned and crisp, breaking it up with a spoon as it cooks.

Step 4 Drain the pasta and place it back in the pan over high heat. Pour in the butternut sauce and toss everything together to thoroughly warm the sauce. Serve in bowls with the crispy sausage mix and fennel fronds on top.

ROLL OF MEXICAN EGG

Preparation time: 5 minutes; cooking time: 10 minutes; servings: 4 2 INGREDIENTS • 1 large egg • a small amount of rapeseed oil for frying • 2 tablespoons tomato salsa • 1 tablespoon fresh coriander

DIRECTIONS

1st Step

1 tbsp water was used to beat the egg. In a medium nonstick pan, heat the oil. Cook until the egg is set, swirling it around the bottom of the pan as if making a pancake. It is not necessary to turn it. Step 2 Carefully place the pancake on a cutting board, spread with salsa, and top with coriander before rolling it up. It can be served hot or cold, and it will keep in the fridge for up to two days.

AUBERGINES MISO

5 minutes to prepare - 50 minutes to cook - 8 servings 2 INGREDIENTS • 2 small aubergines, halved • vegetable oil for roasting and frying • 50g brown miso • 100g giant couscous • 1 red chilli, thinly sliced

DIRECTIONS

1st Step

Preheat the oven to 180°C/160°C fan/gas 4 degrees. Criss-cross the flesh of the aubergines in a diagonal pattern with a sharp knife, then place on a baking tray. 1 tbsp vegetable oil, brushed on the flesh

Step 2 Make a thick paste with the miso and 25ml water. Spread the paste over the aubergines, then cover with foil and roast for 30 minutes in the center of the oven.

Step 3 Remove the foil and continue to roast the aubergines for another 15-20 minutes, or until tender, depending on their size. Step 4 In the meantime, bring a pot of salted water to a boil and heat 1 /2 tbsp vegetable oil in a frying pan over medium-high heat. In a frying pan, toast the couscous for 2 minutes until golden brown, then transfer to a pan of boiling water and cook for 8-10 minutes until tender (or following pack instructions). Drain thoroughly. Serve the aubergines with couscous and a sprinkling of coriander leaves on top.

SWEET POTATO MASH, SESAME SALMON, PURPLE SPROUTING BROCCOLI

Prep time: 10 minutes; cooking time: 15 minutes - Provides food for 1 12 tbsp sesame oil 1 tbsp low-salt soy sauce 2 INGREDIENTS

2 sweet potatoes, scrubbed and cut into wedges • 1 lime, cut into wedges • 2 boneless skinless salmon fillets • 250g purple sprouting broccoli • 1 tbsp sesame seeds • 1 red chilli, thinly sliced (deseeded if you don't like it too hot)

DIRECTIONS

1st Step

Preheat the oven to 200 degrees Celsius/180 degrees Fahrenheit/gas 6 and line a baking tray with parchment paper. Combine 1/2 tbsp sesame oil, soy sauce, ginger, garlic, and honey in a mixing bowl. Toss the sweet potato wedges, skin and all, with the lime wedges in a glass bowl. Microwave on high for 12-14 minutes, or until completely soft, covered in cling film. Step 2 Arrange the broccoli and salmon on the baking tray in the meantime. Season with salt and pepper after spooning over the marinade. Roast for 10-12 minutes in the oven, then top with sesame seeds.

Step 3 Using a fork, roughly mash the sweet potato after removing the lime wedges. Mix in the remaining sesame oil, the chili, and a pinch of salt and pepper. Distribute the salmon and broccoli among the plates.

ADOBO WITH SWEET AND SOUR CHICKEN

In a slow cooker, prepare in 20 minutes and cook for 6 hours and 20 minutes (2 hrs 20 mins on the hob) - Provides food for
INGREDIENTS: 4 INGREDIENTS

• 4 tbsp oil (vegetable)

• 600g skinless boneless chicken thighs, cut in half • 2 tbsp cornflour, plus an extra 1-2 tsp (optional)

• 1 large onion, chopped into chunks • 5 garlic cloves, crushed • 2 red peppers, deseeded and cut into chunks • 400 mL coconut milk • 100 mL low-salt soy sauce • 100 mL white wine vinegar • 50 g soft light brown sugar • 6 bay leaves

DIRECTIONS

Step 1: In a large pan, heat half of the oil. Toss the chicken in a large bowl with the cornflour and season well, then cook in batches until browned all over (don't overcrowd the pan or the chicken won't brown). As you go, pour each batch into the slow cooker, adding a little more oil to the pan if necessary. Cook for a few minutes to soften the onion, garlic, and peppers before adding them to the slow cooker. Step 2 If there's any cornflour left in the bowl, swirl it around with a drop of coconut milk before pouring it into the slow cooker. Season with plenty of black pepper, then add the remaining coconut milk, soy sauce, vinegar, sugar, and bay leaves. Turn the slow cooker to Low, cover, and cook for 5-6 hours, or until the meat is tender and the sauce has thickened. (If you don't have a slow cooker, return the INGREDIENTS to the pan, cover, and cook for 11/2-2 hours, stirring occasionally to avoid sticking and adding a splash of water if the stew appears dry.) If the sauce in the slow cooker is too thin, add the remaining cornflour to thicken it. To thicken the sauce, combine 1-2 teaspoons cornflour with 1-2 teaspoons cold water to make a paste, then ladle 2-3 spoonfuls into a saucepan and bring to a simmer. Stir in the cornflour paste and cook for 1-2 minutes to thicken. Return to the slow cooker and cook for another 10 minutes on High. Serve alongside rice and stir-fried vegetables.

WATERMELON LOLLIES

Prep: 15 minutes Plus at least 4 hours freezing - Serves 6 - 8 INGREDIENTS\s• 1 small watermelon\s• 3 kiwis DIRECTIONS 1.

Halve 1 small watermelon and scrape the flesh out of one half into a dish (you need around 375- 400g) (you need about 375- 400g). Pick out any black seeds. Purée the flesh with a hand blender or in a liquidiser. Fill ice lolly moulds three-quarters full with the purée, put the sticks in if you are using them, and freeze for at least 3 hours, or overnight. Tip any residual purée onto an ice cube tray and freeze it. 2nd Action

Peel 3 kiwis and cut the green meat away from the white center, discarding the core. Purée the flesh. Add a layer of roughly 4-5mm to the top of each lollipop and refreeze for 1 hour. Add some green food colouring to the remainder of the purée to deepen it to the same colour as the watermelon rind.

Pour a very small coating over the top of each lollipop and freeze until you wish to enjoy them.

LAMB DOPIAZA WITH BROCCOLI RICE

Prep: 20 minutes Cook: 1 hour and 30 minutes • THERE ARE ONLY TWO INGREDIENTS IN THIS PRODUCT.

• 225g lamb leg steaks , trimmed with extra fat and sliced into 2.5cm/ 1in chunks\s• 50g full-fat natural bio yogurt , plus 4 tbsp to serve\s• 1 tbsp medium curry powder

• 2 tsp cold-pressed rapeseed oil\s• 2 medium onions , 1 thinly sliced, 1 cut into 5 wedges\s• 2 garlic cloves , peeled and finely sliced\s• 1 tbsp ginger , peeled and finely chopped\s• 1 small red chilli, finely chopped (deseeded if you don't like it too hot)\s• 200g tomatoes , roughly chopped\s• 50g dried split red lentils , rinsed\s• 1/2 small pack of coriander , roughly chopped, plus extra to garnish\s• 100g pack baby leaf spinach

For the broccoli rice\s• 100g wholegrain brown rice\s• 100g tiny broccoli florets

DIRECTIONS

Step 1\sPut the lamb in a large bowl and season generously with ground black pepper. Add the yogurt and 1/ 2 tbsp of the curry powder, and mix well to blend.

Step 2\sHeat half the oil in a large non-stick pot. Fry the onion wedges over a high heat for 4-5 minutes or until nicely browned and slightly soft. Tip onto a platter, put aside and return the pan to the heat.

Step 3\sAdd the remaining oil, the sliced onions, garlic, ginger and chilli, cover and simmer for 10 minutes or until very soft, turning periodically. Remove the top, raise the heat and cook for 2-3 minutes longer or until the onions are tinged with brown – this will add plenty of taste, but make sure they don't become scorched. Step 4\sReduce the heat once again and toss in the tomatoes and remaining curry powder.

Simmer for 1 min, then pour the lamb and yogurt into the pan and cook over a medium-high heat for 4-5 minutes, stirring occasionally. Step 5\sPour 300ml cold water into the pan, toss in the lentils and coriander, cover with a lid and let to cook over a low heat for 45 minutes - the sauce should be simmering gently and you may add a splash of water if the curry becomes a little dry. Remove the cover every 10-15 minutes and stir the curry. Step 6\sWith half an hour of the curry cooking time left, cook the rice in plenty of boiling water for 25 minutes or until just tender. Add the broccoli florets and simmer for a further 3 minutes. Well-drained

Step 7

Remove the cover from the curry, add the saved onion wedges and continue to simmer over a high heat for a further 15 minutes or until the lamb is cooked, stirring constantly. Just before serving, toss in the spinach, a handful at a time, and allow it wilt. Serve with the yogurt, coriander and broccoli rice.

CHARGRILLED CHICKEN & KALE CAESAR SALAD

Prep: 20 minutes - Cook: 20 mins • 4 INGREDIENTS\s• 1 anchovy\s• 1 garlic clove\s• 1 tsp Dijon mustard\s• 100ml buttermilk\s• 1 lemon , zested and juiced\s• 200g bag kale , large tough stalks removed\s• 200g defrosted frozen peas\s• 6 skinless and boneless chicken thighs\s• 2 thick slices crusty bread\s• 3 tbsp cold pressed rapeseed oil\s• 400g long-stem broccoli , cut in half lengthways\s• 30g parmesan DIRECTIONS Step 1\sMash the anchovy and garlic together using a pestle and mortar, then transfer the mixture into a bowl and whisk in the mustard, buttermilk, lemon zest and juice, and season with black pepper. Put the kale and peas in a big bowl, pour over ¾ of the dressing, then massage into the greens so each leaf is covered. Step 2\sPut the chicken thighs between two sheets of baking paper, then smash out with a rolling pin to 1cm thickness.

Step 3\sHeat a griddle pan until scorching hot. Brush the bread pieces with a little oil, then fry until gently browned on both sides. Set aside.

Step 4\sNext, season the broccoli and brush the cut side of each piece with a little oil. Griddle, cut-side down, in batches for 3-4 minutes until tender. Lastly, spray the remaining oil over the chicken thighs and season, then griddle the chicken for 3-4 minutes on each side until cooked through.

Step 5\sDistribute the greens amongst four dishes. Slice the chicken diagonally and cut the bread into pieces. Top each of the dishes with ¼ of the chicken, broccoli and croutons.

Grate over the parmesan in big shavings and sprinkle with the remaining dressing to serve.

SLOW COOKER TURKISH BREAKFAST EGGS

Prep: 15 minutes - Cook: 5 hours - 6 hrs • THERE ARE FOUR INGREDIENTS IN THIS PRODUCT.

• 1 tbsp olive oil\s• 2 onions , finely sliced\s• 1 red pepper , cored and finely sliced\s• 1 small red chilli , finely sliced\s• 8 cherry tomatoes\s• 1 slice sourdough bread , cubed\s• 4 eggs\s• 2 tbsp skimmed milk\s• small bunch parsley , finely chopped\s• 4 tbsp natural yogurt , to serve

DIRECTIONS

1.

Oil the interior of a small slow cooker and heat if required. Heat the remaining oil in a heavy- based frying pan. Stir in the onions, pepper and chilli. Cook until they begin to soften. Tip into the slow cooker and add the cherry tomatoes and bread and mix everything. Season.

Step 2\sWhisk the eggs with the milk and parsley and pour this over the top, ensuring sure all the other INGREDIENTS are coated. Cook for 5-6 hours. Serve with the yogurt.

PRAWN FRIED RICE

Prep: 5 minutes - Cook: 25 mins |

Serves 4 INGREDIENTS\s• 250g long-grain brown rice\s• 150g frozen peas\s• 100g mangetout\s• 1½ tbsp rapeseed oil\s• 1 onion , finely chopped\s• 2 garlic cloves , crushed\s• thumb-sized piece of ginger , finely grated\s• 150g raw king prawns\s• 3 medium eggs , beaten\s• 2 tsp sesame seeds\s• 1 tbsp low-salt soy sauce

• ½ tbsp rice or white wine vinegar\s• 4 spring onions , trimmed and sliced

DIRECTIONS

1.

Cook the rice following box directions. Boil a separate pan of water and blanch the peas and mangetout for 1 min, then drain and put aside with the rice.

2nd Action

Meanwhile, heat the oil in a large non-stick frying pan or wok over a medium heat and cook the onion for 10 minutes or until golden brown. Add the garlic and ginger and cook for a further minute. Tip in the blanched veggies and cook for 5 minutes, then the prawns and fry for a further 2 mins. Stir the rice into the pan then put everything to one side. Pour the beaten eggs into the empty side of the pan and swirl to scramble them. Fold everything together with the sesame seeds, soy and vinegar, then finish with the spring onions distributed over.

HAM & PICCALILLI SALAD

Prep: 15 minutes - No cook - Serves 4 INGREDIENTS\s• 4 tbsp piccalilli\s• 3 tbsp natural yogurt

• 12 silverskin pickled onions , halved\s• 130g pea shoots\s• 180g pulled ham hock or shredded cooked ham\s• ½ cucumber , halved and thinly sliced\s• 100g fresh peas\s• 40g mature cheddar , shaved\s• crusty bread , to serve

DIRECTIONS

Step 1\sMix the piccalilli, yogurt, onions and 4 tbsp water together to produce a dressing. Season and put away. Step 2\sToss the pea shoots, ham, cucumber and peas together.

Pile onto a serving platter, then drizzle over the dressing. Top with the cheese and serve with crusty bread.

AVOCADO & BEAN TRIANGLES

Prep: 5 minutes - No cook |

Serves 2 INGREDIENTS\s• 3 triangluar bread thins\s• 210g can red kidney beans , drained\s• 1 tbsp finely chopped dill , plus extra for garnish\s• 1/2 lemon , for squeezing\s• 1 tomato , diced\s• 1 small avocado\s• 1 small red onion , roughly chopped

DIRECTIONS

Step 1\sFollow our triangle bread thins recipe to create your own. While they bake, coarsely mash the beans with the dill and a big squeeze of lemon then toss in the tomato.

Step 2\sCut the bread triangles in half and top with the beans. Scoop the avocado into a bowl and coarsely mash with a squeeze more lemon. Spoon the avocado atop the beans, sprinkle over the chopped onion, then garnish with the remaining dill.

SUMMER CARROT, TARRAGON & WHITE BEAN SOUP

10 minutes to prepare - 20 minutes to cook • 4
INGREDIENTS\s• 1 tbsp rapeseed oil\s• 2 large leeks , well
washed, halved lengthways and finely sliced\s• 700g carrots ,
chopped\s• 1.4l hot reduced-salt vegetable bouillon (we used
Marigold)\s• 4 garlic cloves , finely grated\s• 2 x 400g cans
cannellini beans in water\s• ⅔ small pack tarragon , leaves
roughly chopped

DIRECTIONS

1.

Heat the oil over a medium heat in a big pan and cook the
leeks and carrots for 5 minutes to soften.

Step 2\sPour over the stock, toss in the garlic, the beans with
their liquid, and three-quarters of the tarragon, then cover
and cook for 15 minutes or until the veg is just soft. Stir in the
remaining tarragon before serving.

WHITE VELVET SOUP WITH SMOKY ALMONDS

10 minutes to prepare - 25 minutes to cook • 2
INGREDIENTS\s• 2 tsp rapeseed oil\s• 2 big garlic cloves ,
sliced\s• 2 leeks, cut so they're primarily white in colour,

rinsed carefully, then sliced (approximately 240g)\s• 200g cauliflower , chopped\s• 2 tsp vegetable bouillon powder

• 400g cannellini beans , rinsed\s• fresh nutmeg , for grating\s• 100ml whole milk\s• 25g whole almonds , chopped\s• ½ tsp smoky paprika

• 2 x 25g slices rye bread , to serve

DIRECTIONS

Step 1\sHeat the oil in a big pan. Add the garlic, leeks and cauliflower and simmer for approximately 5 minutes, turning constantly, until beginning to soften (but not browning) (but not colouring).

Step 2\sStir in the vegetable bouillon and beans, pour in 600ml boiling water and add a few generous gratings of the nutmeg. Cover and allow to boil for 15 minutes until the leeks and cauliflower are soft. Add the milk and whiz with a hand blender until smooth and creamy.

Step 3\sPut the almonds in a dry pan and simmer very gently for 1 min, or until toasted, then remove from the heat. Scatter the paprika over the almonds and stir thoroughly.

Ladle the soup into bowls, sprinkle with the spicy nuts and serve with the rye bread.

POLISH APPLE CAKE (SZARLOTKA) (SZARLOTKA)

Prep: 35 minutes - Cook: 1 hour + freezing • THE INGREDIENTS ARE AS FOLLOWS: 12 INSTRUCTIONS

For the filling\s• half a lemon

• 4 tbsp light brown sugar • 1 tbsp crushed cinnamon • 6 big Bramley or cooking apples

For the dough\s• 450g plain flour , plus additional for dusting\s• 1 tsp baking powder

• 225g golden caster sugar • 200g unsalted butter, cut into pieces, plus extra for greasing • 3 egg yolks, plus 1 whole egg, at room temperature • 1 tbsp natural yogurt

• 1 teaspoon lemon zest (from half a lemon) • 1 teaspoon vanilla extract

assisting

• icing sugar • 300ml pot whipping cream • 1 teaspoon cinnamon DIRECTIONS 1.

Preheat the oven to 180°C/160°C fan/gas mark 4 4. Using baking paper, grease and line a 20 x 29cm baking pan. Step 2 Zest half a lemon for the filling and set aside for the dough. To keep the apples from browning, peel, core, and thinly slice them, then pour over the lemon juice. In a large saucepan, combine the apples, sugar, 200ml water, and cinnamon. Cook for 5 minutes, then remove from the heat and chill in the liquid (this will come in handy later).

Step 3 To prepare the dough, pulse or whisk together the flour and baking powder in a food processor or a large mixing bowl. Mix in the butter until the mixture resembles sand. To make a dough, combine the sugar, egg yolks, and egg, yogurt, lemon zest, and vanilla essence. Place it on a floured surface to cool. Roll it into a ball by bringing it together with your hands.

Step 4: Cut the dough in half, cover one side in plastic wrap, and place in the freezer for 1 hour. The remaining half of the dough should be rolled out large enough to fill the bottom of the lined pan. Push the dough halfway up the edges of the tray with the palm of your hand until the whole base is covered. Prick the dough all over with a fork and bake for 15 minutes, or until brown and springy to the touch.

Step 5 Spoon nearly half of the cooking liquid over the apple filling, then put aside.

6th step

Take the dough out of the freezer and roughly grate it like a block of cheese. Sprinkle the grated dough over the apples and bake for 40-45 minutes, or until the topping is brown and the apples are tender. Allow it cool fully before cutting into squares and dusting with icing sugar. Whip the cream until stiff, then fold in the cinnamon and serve with the cake.

BOLOGNESE VEGAN

Preparation time: 20 minutes; cooking time: 1 hour; servings: 6 INGREDIENTS: 3

• 15g dried porcini mushrooms • 1 12 tbsp olive oil • 12 onion, finely chopped • 1 carrot, finely chopped • 1 celery stick, finely chopped • 2 garlic cloves, sliced • 2 thyme sprigs • 12 tsp tomato purée • 50ml vegan red wine (optional) • 125g dried green lentils • 400g can whole plum tomatoes • 125g chestnut mushrooms, chopped

DIRECTIONS

1.

Pour 400ml boiling water over the dried porcini and let aside for 10 minutes to allow the porcini to absorb the water. In a big pot, add 1 tablespoon of oil. Toss in the onion, carrot, and celery, as well as a sprinkle of salt. Cook for 10 minutes, stirring occasionally, until soft. Remove the porcini from the liquid, reserving the mushroomy stock, and coarsely chop the porcini. Set one aside and the other aside.

Step 2 In the same pan, add the garlic and thyme. Cook for 1 minute before adding the tomato purée and cooking for another minute. If using, add the red wine and heat until almost reduced before adding the lentils, saved mushroom stock, and tomatoes. Bring to a boil, then lower to a low heat and cover to keep it warm.

Step 3 Preheat a big frying pan in the meanwhile. After that, add the chestnut, portobello, and rehydrated mushrooms, along with the remaining oil. Fry until all of the liquid has drained and the mushrooms have become a rich golden brown color. Add the soy sauce and mix well. Scrape the mushrooms into the lentil mixture after thoroughly mixing everything. 4)

Stir in the Marmite and boil the ragu over a low-medium heat, stirring periodically, for 30-45 minutes, or until the lentils are cooked and the sauce is thick and reduced, adding more water if required. Remove the thyme sprigs and season with salt and pepper to taste.

Step 5 Boil the spaghetti for 1 minute less than the package instructions in a large pot of salted water. Drain the pasta, reserving a ladleful of the water, then toss the spaghetti in the sauce, loosening up the ragu slightly with a little of the starchy liquid so the pasta clings to the sauce. Serve with a sprinkle of black pepper and fresh basil.

ROSES WITH SUGAR

1 hr total time Each batch takes 1 hour. a lack of a cook Roses and leaves for 40 roses INGREDIENTS

a paste that can be eaten 200g ready-to-roll icing, plus a small amount of solid vegetable fat for rolling optional edible sparkles (we used bright pink), optional edible lustre (we used a shimmery pink), optional edible lustre (we used a shimmery pink), optional edible lustre (we used a shimmery pink), optional edible

DIRECTIONS

1.

Begin with the roses and work your way up from there. Knead a small amount of the color paste into 150g of icing until it is pale and even. Break the dough into three balls, then add a little more color to two of them to create three different color depths. Wrap in cling film and store in a cool, dry place. Over a smooth work surface, rub a very thin layer of fat. One of the icing balls should be rolled out thinly (about 1-2mm) and cut into an 8 x 20cm rectangle. Cut a 1cm wide strip of icing from the rest of the icing.

Step 2 Roll the icing carefully up and around itself. Start rolling slightly skew-whiff so that the finished rose's outside edge sticks out further than the middle for a more realistic rose appearance. Begin guiding the end of the icing down and under to form a neat rosebud with about 2cm to go.

Cut or pinch off the bottom after pinching to shape. Allow at least 1 hour for the mixture to firm up. Using the remaining icing, repeat the procedure.

Color the remaining icing green for the leaves. Pinch off pea-size pieces, roll into balls, and flatten slightly. Make a leaf by pinching one end. Allow to air dry before using.

4)

Dust a little lustre onto each rose with a paintbrush or your fingertip once the roses have dried and firmed up. If desired, add a few sparkles. Arrange three roses in a cluster on each cupcake, then three leaves. To make 12 cakes, you'll need 36 roses and leaves.

SMOOOTHIE WITH AVOCADO AND STRAWBERRY

5 minutes to prepare - no cooking required - serves 6 12 avocado, stoned, peeled, and cut into chunks • 150g strawberry, halved • 4 tbsp low-fat natural yogurt

• 200 mL semi-skimmed milk • lemon or lime juice, to taste DIRECTIONS 1.

Blend all of the ingredients until smooth in a blender. Add a little water if the mixture is too thick.

PIE WITH SAMOSA

5 minutes to prepare – 30 minutes to cook • • 2-3 tbsp vegetable oil • 1 chopped onion • 500g lamb mince • 2 finely chopped garlic cloves • 2 tbsp curry powder

• 1 large peeled and grated sweet potato (approximately 300g) • 100g frozen peas • 1 handful coarsely chopped coriander

• 1 tsp cumin seeds • 3-4 sheets filo pastry DIRECTIONS 1.

Preheat the oven to 180 degrees Fahrenheit/160 degrees Fahrenheit fan/gas 3. 4. In a frying pan, warm 1 tablespoon of oil. Cook for 5 minutes, or until the meat is browned, with the onion and mince. Add the garlic, curry powder, sweet potato, and 300ml water and stir to combine. Cook until the potato is soft, about 5-8 minutes. Season with salt and pepper after adding the peas, coriander, and lemon juice.

Step 2 Transfer the batter to a baking dish. Scrunch the filo sheets over the top of the mince, brushing with the remaining oil. Bake for 10-15 minutes, or until the top is crisp, sprinkled with cumin seeds.

BRLÉE TART WITH GOOSEBERRY CREAM

10 minute prep time - 1 hour and 20 minute cook time • 8 INGREDIENTS • 450g gooseberries • 200g white caster sugar • 4 eggs • 100ml double cream • 500g block sweet pastry DIRECTIONS Step 1 Combine the gooseberries, 100 grams of sugar, and 100 milliliters of water in a saucepan. Cook for 8-

10 minutes, or until the fruit is soft and the juices have thickened into a syrup. Place the fruit in a sieve over a jug and strain the syrupy juices; you'll need about 150ml. Fill a bowl halfway with the pulp and set it aside to cool.

Step 2 Whisk together the eggs and 50g of sugar in a separate bowl, then add the cream and gooseberry syrup. Set aside after straining through a sieve into a new jug.

Step 3 Preheat the oven to 160 degrees Fahrenheit/140 degrees Fahrenheit fan/gas 3. 3. Roll out the pastry to the thickness of a £1 coin on a lightly floured surface, then transfer to a 23cm tart pan. Gently press the bottom and sides together, leaving a small overhang. Fill the tart with baking beans and cover with foil. After 10 minutes, remove the foil and beans and continue baking for another 20 minutes. Allow to cool after removing from the oven.

Step 4 Lower the temperature of the oven to 150°C/130°C fan/gas. 2. Evenly spread the pulp over the tart's base, then carefully pour the cream mixture over it to make two layers. Bake for 35-40 minutes, or until the cream layer wobbles a little. Trim the pastry edges after removing it from the oven. Allow to cool completely before scattering the remaining sugar on top and caramelizing with a blowtorch if desired. Serve immediately.

MASALA TIKKA WITH RED PEPPER AND BEANS

10 minutes to prepare - 20 minutes to cook • 2 INGREDIENTS • 1 tbsp vegetable oil • 1 onion, chopped • 2 red peppers, deseeded and cut into strips • 1 garlic clove, crushed • thumb-sized piece of ginger, grated • 1 red chilli, finely chopped

DIRECTIONS

1.

In a medium saucepan, heat the oil, then add the onion and red peppers, along with a pinch of salt, and cook for about 5 minutes, until softened. Tip in the garlic, ginger and red chilli along with the spices and fry for a couple of mins longer.

Step 2\sSpoon in the tomato purée, stir, then tip in the baked beans along with 100ml water. Bubble for 5 mins, then squeeze in the lemon juice. Serve with the rice and scatter over the coriander leaves.

BASIC CURRIED ROAST CHICKPEAS

5 minutes to prepare – 20 minutes to cook • 4 INGREDIENTS\s• 2 x 400g cans chickpeas\s• 1½ tbsp

rapeseed oil\s• 1 tsp caraway seeds\s• 1 tsp mustard seeds\s• 1 tbsp curry powder

DIRECTIONS

1.

Preheat the oven to 200 degrees Fahrenheit/180 degrees Fahrenheit fan/gas 6. 6. Drain the chickpeas and pat with a tea towel to remove as much moisture as possible. Tip them onto a roasting tray, toss with the oil, seeds and seasoning and roast for 20 mins until golden brown. Toss in the curry powder and enjoy.

LENTIL & CAULIFLOWER CURRY

Prep: 10 mins - Cook: 40 mins - Serves 4 INGREDIENTS

• 1 tbsp olive oil\s• 1 large onion, chopped\s• 3 tbsp curry paste\s• 1 tsp turmeric\s• 1 tsp mustard seeds\s• 200g red or yellow lentil\s• 1l low-sodium vegetable or chicken stock (made with 2 cubes)\s• 1 large cauliflower, broken into florets\s• 1 large potato, diced\s• 3 tbsp coconut yogurt

• small pack coriander, chopped\s• juice 1 lemon

• 100g cooked brown rice

DIRECTIONS

1.

Heat the oil in a large saucepan and cook the onion until soft, about 5 mins. Add the curry paste, spices and lentils, then stir to coat the lentils in the onions and paste. Pour over the stock and simmer for 20 mins, then add the cauliflower, potato and a little extra water if it looks a bit dry. Step 2\sSimmer for about 12 mins until the cauliflower and potatoes are tender. Stir in the yogurt, coriander and lemon juice, and serve with the brown rice.

SPICY CHICKEN & BEAN STEW

Prep: 15 mins - Cook: 1 hr and 20 mins • 6 INGREDIENTS

• 1¼ kg chicken thighs and drumsticks (approx. weight, we used a 1.23kg mixed pack)\s• 1 tbsp olive oil\s• 2 onions, sliced\s• 1 garlic clove, crushed\s• 2 red chillies, deseeded and chopped\s• 250g frozen peppers, defrosted\s• 400g can chopped tomatoes\s• 420g can kidney beans in chilli sauce

• 2 x 400g cans butter beans, drained\s• 400ml hot chicken stock\s• small bunch coriander, chopped\s• 150ml pot soured cream and crusty bread, to serve

DIRECTIONS

Step 1\sPull the skin off the chicken and discard. Heat the oil in a large casserole dish, brown the chicken all over, then remove with a slotted spoon. Tip in the onions, garlic and chillies, then fry for 5 mins until starting to soften and turn golden.

Step 2\sAdd the peppers, tomatoes, beans and hot stock. Put the chicken back on top, half-cover with a pan lid and cook for 50 mins, until the chicken is cooked through and tender.

Step 3\sStir through the coriander and serve with soured cream and crusty bread.

ORANGE & RASPBERRY GRANOLA

Prep: 15 mins - Cook: 25 mins plus at least 1 hr chilling • THERE ARE FOUR INGREDIENTS IN THIS PRODUCT.

• 400g jumbo oats\s• juice 2 oranges (150ml), plus zest of 1/2

• 1 tsp ground cinnamon

• 2 tbsp freeze-dried raspberries or strawberries (see tip)\s•
25g flaked almonds , toasted\s• 25g mixed seeds (such as
sunflower, pumpkin, sesame and linseed) (such as sunflower,
pumpkin, sesame and linseed)

assisting

• 2 large oranges , peeled and segmented\s• mint leaves
(optional) (optional)

DIRECTIONS

1.

Put 200g oats and 500ml water in a food processor and blitz
for 1 min. Line a sieve with clean muslin and pour in the oat
mixture. Leave to drip through for 5 mins, then twist the
ends of the muslin and squeeze well to capture as much of
the oat milk as possible– it should be the consistency of
single cream. Best chilled at least 1 hr before serving. Can be
kept in a sealed or covered jug in the fridge for up to 3 days.
Step 2\sHeat oven to 200C/180C fan/gas 6 and line a baking
tray with baking parchment. Put the orange juice in a
medium saucepan and bring to the boil. Boil rapidly for 5

mins or until the liquid has reduced by half, stirring occasionally. Mix the remaining 200g oats with the orange zest and cinnamon. Remove the pan from the heat and stir the oat mixture into the juice. Spread over the lined tray in a thin layer and bake for 10-15 mins or until lightly browned and crisp, turning the oats every few mins. Leave to cool on the tray. 3rd Action

Once cool, mix the oats with the raspberries, flaked almonds and seeds. Can be kept in a sealed jar for up to one week. To serve, spoon the granola into bowls, pour over the oat milk and top with the orange segments and mint leaves, if you like.

HERBY CHICKEN GYROS

Prep: 10 mins - Cook: 4 mins - Serves 2 INGREDIENTS\s• 1 large skinless chicken breast\s• rapeseed oil , for brushing\s• small garlic clove , crushed\s• ½ tsp dried oregano\s• 2 tbsp Greek yogurt

• 10 cm piece cucumber , grated, excess juice squeezed out\s• 2 tbsp chopped mint , plus a few leaves to serve\s• 2 wholemeal pitta breads\s• 2 red or yellow tomatoes , sliced\s• 1 red pepper from a jar (not in oil), deseeded and sliced

DIRECTIONS

1.

Cut the chicken breast in half lengthways, then cover with cling film and bash with a rolling pin to flatten it. Brush with some oil, then cover with the garlic, oregano and some pepper. Heat a non-stick frying pan and cook the chicken for a few mins each side. Meanwhile, mix the yogurt, cucumber and mint to make tzatziki. 2nd Action

Cut the tops from the pittas along their longest side and stuff with the chicken, tomato, pepper and tzatziki. Poke in a few mint leaves to serve. If taking to the office for lunch, pack the tzatziki in a separate pot and add just before eating to prevent the pitta going soggy before lunchtime.

ROAST ROOTS WITH GOAT'S CHEESE & SPINACH

Prep: 30 mins - Cook: 55 mins • THERE ARE ONLY TWO INGREDIENTS IN THIS PRODUCT.

• 350g butternut squash , deseeded and cut into chunks, peeled if you like • 200g carrots , peeled and cut into long batons • 250g parsnips , peeled and cut into long batons • 200g raw beetroot , well-scrubbed and cut into thick wedges

• 1 medium red onion , cut into wedges

• 1 tbsp cold-pressed rapeseed oil • juice and finely grated zest 1 citrus fruit

• 1 bulb garlic , cloves separated • 4-5 thyme sprigs , leaves roughly chopped • 75g soft rindless goat's cheese log • 25g mixed nuts , such as brazils, almonds, hazelnuts, pecans and walnuts, roughly chopped • 50g baby leaf spinach

DIRECTIONS

1.

Preheat the oven to 200 degrees Fahrenheit/180 degrees Fahrenheit fan/gas 6. 6. Put the vegetables, without the garlic, into a bowl and toss with the oil, lemon zest and juice and plenty of ground black pepper.

Step 2 Scatter the vegetables over a large baking tray or roasting tin and bake for 30 mins. Take the tray out of the oven, add the garlic and thyme, then turn the vegetables. Return to the oven for 20 mins or until the vegetables are tender and lightly browned, turning halfway through. Dot with the goat's cheese and nuts, scatter over the spinach and return to the oven for 3-5 mins or until the spinach has wilted and the goat's cheese has begun to melt. You can press the softened garlic cloves out of their skins and mash with the roasted vegetables, if you like.

SPICE-CRUSTED AUBERGINES & PEPPERS WITH PILAF

10 minutes to prepare - 30 minutes to cook • 4 INGREDIENTS • 2 large aubergines , halved • 2 tbsp extra virgin olive oil • 2 red peppers , quartered • 2 tsp ground cinnamon • 2 tsp chilli flakes • 2 tsp za'atar • 4 tbsp pomegranate molasses • 140g puy lentils • 140g basmati rice • seeds from 1 pomegranate • small pack flat-leaf parsley , roughly chopped • Greek or coconut yogurt , to serve

DIRECTIONS

1.

Preheat oven to 220 degrees Celsius/200 degrees Celsius fan/gas 7. Using a sharp knife, score a diamond pattern into the aubergines. Brush with 1 tbsp of the oil, season well and place on a baking tray, cut-side down. Cook in the oven for 15 mins. Add the peppers to the tray, turn the aubergines over and drizzle everything with the remaining oil. Sprinkle over the spices, 1 tbsp of the pomegranate molasses and a little salt. Roast in the oven for 15 mins more. Step 2 Boil the lentils in plenty of water until al dente. After they've been boiling for 5 mins, add the rice. Cook for 10 mins or until cooked through but with a bit of bite. Drain and return to the pan, covered with a lid to keep warm.

3rd Action

Stir the pomegranate seeds and parsley through the lentil rice. Divide between four plates or tip onto a large platter. Top with the roasted veg, a dollop of yogurt and the remaining pomegranate molasses drizzled over.

POTATO PANCAKES WITH CHARD & EGGS

10 minutes to prepare - 15 minutes to cook • 2 INGREDIENTS • 300g mashed potato • 4 spring onions , very finely chopped • 25g plain wholemeal flour • ½ tsp baking powder • 3 eggs • 2 tsp rapeseed oil • 240g chard , stalks and leaves roughly chopped, or baby spinach, chopped

DIRECTIONS

Step 1 Mix the mash, spring onions, flour, baking powder and 1 of the eggs in a bowl. Heat the oil in a non-stick frying pan, then spoon in the potato mix to make two mounds. Flatten them to form two 15cm discs and fry for 5-8 mins until the undersides are set and golden, then carefully ip over and cook on the other side. Step 2 Meanwhile, wash the chard and put in a pan with some of the water still clinging to it, then cover and cook over a medium heat for 5 mins until wilted and tender. Poach the remaining eggs.

Step 3 Top the pancakes with the greens and egg. Serve while the yolks are still runny.Step 5 Boil the spaghetti for 1 minute less than the package instructions in a large pot of salted water. Drain the pasta, reserving a ladleful of the water, then toss the spaghetti in the sauce, loosening up the ragu slightly with a little of the starchy liquid so the pasta clings to the sauce. Serve with a sprinkle of black pepper and fresh basil.

ROSES WITH SUGAR

1 hr total time Each batch takes 1 hour. a lack of a cook Roses and leaves for 40 roses INGREDIENTS

a paste that can be eaten 200g ready-to-roll icing, plus a small amount of solid vegetable fat for rolling optional edible sparkles (we used bright pink), optional edible lustre (we used a shimmery pink), optional edible lustre (we used a shimmery pink), optional edible lustre (we used a shimmery pink), optional edible

DIRECTIONS

1.

Begin with the roses and work your way up from there. Knead a small amount of the color paste into 150g of icing until it is pale and even. Break the dough into three balls, then add a little more color to two of them to create three different color depths. Wrap in cling film and store in a cool, dry place. Over a smooth work surface, rub a very thin layer of fat. One of the icing balls should be rolled out thinly (about 1-2mm) and cut into an 8 x 20cm rectangle. Cut a 1cm wide strip of icing from the rest of the icing.

Step 2 Roll the icing carefully up and around itself. Start rolling slightly skew-whiff so that the finished rose's outside edge sticks out further than the middle for a more realistic rose appearance. Begin guiding the end of the icing down and under to form a neat rosebud with about 2cm to go.

Cut or pinch off the bottom after pinching to shape. Allow at least 1 hour for the mixture to firm up. Using the remaining icing, repeat the procedure.

Color the remaining icing green for the leaves. Pinch off pea-size pieces, roll into balls, and flatten slightly. Make a leaf by pinching one end. Allow to air dry before using.

4)

Dust a little lustre onto each rose with a paintbrush or your fingertip once the roses have dried and firmed up. If desired, add a few sparkles. Arrange three roses in a cluster on each cupcake, then three leaves. To make 12 cakes, you'll need 36 roses and leaves.

SMOOOTHIE WITH AVOCADO AND STRAWBERRY

5 minutes to prepare - no cooking required - serves 6 12 avocado, stoned, peeled, and cut into chunks • 150g strawberry, halved • 4 tbsp low-fat natural yogurt

• 200 mL semi-skimmed milk • lemon or lime juice, to taste DIRECTIONS 1.

Blend all of the ingredients until smooth in a blender. Add a little water if the mixture is too thick.

PIE WITH SAMOSA

5 minutes to prepare – 30 minutes to cook • • 2-3 tbsp vegetable oil • 1 chopped onion • 500g lamb mince • 2 finely

chopped garlic cloves • 2 tbsp curry powder

• 1 large peeled and grated sweet potato (approximately 300g) • 100g frozen peas • 1 handful coarsely chopped coriander

• 1 tsp cumin seeds • 3-4 sheets filo pastry DIRECTIONS 1.

Preheat the oven to 180 degrees Fahrenheit/160 degrees Fahrenheit fan/gas 3. 4. In a frying pan, warm 1 tablespoon of oil. Cook for 5 minutes, or until the meat is browned, with the onion and mince. Add the garlic, curry powder, sweet potato, and 300ml water and stir to combine. Cook until the potato is soft, about 5-8 minutes. Season with salt and pepper after adding the peas, coriander, and lemon juice.

Step 2 Transfer the batter to a baking dish. Scrunch the filo sheets over the top of the mince, brushing with the remaining oil. Bake for 10-15 minutes, or until the top is crisp, sprinkled with cumin seeds.

BRLÉE TART WITH GOOSEBERRY CREAM

10 minute prep time - 1 hour and 20 minute cook time • 8 INGREDIENTS • 450g gooseberries • 200g white caster sugar • 4 eggs • 100ml double cream • 500g block sweet pastry

DIRECTIONS Step 1 Combine the gooseberries, 100 grams of sugar, and 100 milliliters of water in a saucepan. Cook for 8-10 minutes, or until the fruit is soft and the juices have thickened into a syrup. Place the fruit in a sieve over a jug and strain the syrupy juices; you'll need about 150ml. Fill a bowl halfway with the pulp and set it aside to cool.

Step 2 Whisk together the eggs and 50g of sugar in a separate bowl, then add the cream and gooseberry syrup. Set aside after straining through a sieve into a new jug.

Step 3 Preheat the oven to 160 degrees Fahrenheit/140 degrees Fahrenheit fan/gas 3. 3. Roll out the pastry to the thickness of a £1 coin on a lightly floured surface, then transfer to a 23cm tart pan. Gently press the bottom and sides together, leaving a small overhang. Fill the tart with baking beans and cover with foil. After 10 minutes, remove the foil and beans and continue baking for another 20 minutes. Allow to cool after removing from the oven.

Step 4 Lower the temperature of the oven to 150°C/130°C fan/gas. 2. Evenly spread the pulp over the tart's base, then carefully pour the cream mixture over it to make two layers. Bake for 35-40 minutes, or until the cream layer wobbles a little. Trim the pastry edges after removing it from the oven. Allow to cool completely before scattering the remaining sugar on top and caramelizing with a blowtorch if desired. Serve immediately.

MASALA TIKKA WITH RED PEPPER AND BEANS

10 minutes to prepare - 20 minutes to cook • 2 INGREDIENTS • 1 tbsp vegetable oil • 1 onion, chopped • 2 red peppers, deseeded and cut into strips • 1 garlic clove, crushed • thumb-sized piece of ginger, grated • 1 red chilli, finely chopped

DIRECTIONS

1.

In a medium saucepan, heat the oil, then add the onion and red peppers, along with a pinch of salt, and cook for about 5 minutes, until softened. Tip in the garlic, ginger and red chilli along with the spices and fry for a couple of mins longer.

Step 2\sSpoon in the tomato purée, stir, then tip in the baked beans along with 100ml water. Bubble for 5 mins, then squeeze in the lemon juice. Serve with the rice and scatter over the coriander leaves.

BASIC CURRIED ROAST CHICKPEAS

5 minutes to prepare – 20 minutes to cook • 4 INGREDIENTS\s• 2 x 400g cans chickpeas\s• 1½ tbsp rapeseed oil\s• 1 tsp caraway seeds\s• 1 tsp mustard seeds\s• 1 tbsp curry powder

DIRECTIONS

1.

Preheat the oven to 200 degrees Fahrenheit/180 degrees Fahrenheit fan/gas 6. 6. Drain the chickpeas and pat with a tea towel to remove as much moisture as possible. Tip them onto a roasting tray, toss with the oil, seeds and seasoning and roast for 20 mins until golden brown. Toss in the curry powder and enjoy.

LENTIL & CAULIFLOWER CURRY

Prep: 10 mins - Cook: 40 mins - Serves 4 INGREDIENTS

• 1 tbsp olive oil\s• 1 large onion, chopped\s• 3 tbsp curry paste\s• 1 tsp turmeric\s• 1 tsp mustard seeds\s• 200g red or yellow lentil\s• 1l low-sodium vegetable or chicken stock (made with 2 cubes)\s• 1 large cauliflower, broken into florets\s• 1 large potato, diced\s• 3 tbsp coconut yogurt

• small pack coriander, chopped\s• juice 1 lemon

• 100g cooked brown rice

DIRECTIONS

1.

Heat the oil in a large saucepan and cook the onion until soft, about 5 mins. Add the curry paste, spices and lentils, then stir to coat the lentils in the onions and paste. Pour over the stock and simmer for 20 mins, then add the cauliflower, potato and a little extra water if it looks a bit dry. Step 2\sSimmer for about 12 mins until the cauliflower and potatoes are tender. Stir in the yogurt, coriander and lemon juice, and serve with the brown rice.

SPICY CHICKEN & BEAN STEW

Prep: 15 mins - Cook: 1 hr and 20 mins • 6 INGREDIENTS

• 1¼ kg chicken thighs and drumsticks (approx. weight, we used a 1.23kg mixed pack)\s• 1 tbsp olive oil\s• 2 onions, sliced\s• 1 garlic clove, crushed\s• 2 red chillies, deseeded and chopped\s• 250g frozen peppers, defrosted\s• 400g can chopped tomatoes\s• 420g can kidney beans in chilli sauce

• 2 x 400g cans butter beans, drained\s• 400ml hot chicken stock\s• small bunch coriander, chopped\s• 150ml pot soured cream and crusty bread, to serve

DIRECTIONS

Step 1\sPull the skin off the chicken and discard. Heat the oil in a large casserole dish, brown the chicken all over, then remove with a slotted spoon. Tip in the onions, garlic and chillies, then fry for 5 mins until starting to soften and turn golden.

Step 2\sAdd the peppers, tomatoes, beans and hot stock. Put the chicken back on top, half-cover with a pan lid and cook for 50 mins, until the chicken is cooked through and tender.

Step 3\sStir through the coriander and serve with soured cream and crusty bread.

ORANGE & RASPBERRY GRANOLA

Prep: 15 mins - Cook: 25 mins plus at least 1 hr chilling • THERE ARE FOUR INGREDIENTS IN THIS PRODUCT.

• 400g jumbo oats\s• juice 2 oranges (150ml), plus zest of 1/2

• 1 tsp ground cinnamon

• 2 tbsp freeze-dried raspberries or strawberries (see tip)\s• 25g flaked almonds , toasted\s• 25g mixed seeds (such as sunflower, pumpkin, sesame and linseed) (such as sunflower, pumpkin, sesame and linseed)

assisting

• 2 large oranges , peeled and segmented\s• mint leaves (optional) (optional)

DIRECTIONS

1.

Put 200g oats and 500ml water in a food processor and blitz for 1 min. Line a sieve with clean muslin and pour in the oat mixture. Leave to drip through for 5 mins, then twist the ends of the muslin and squeeze well to capture as much of the oat milk as possible– it should be the consistency of single cream. Best chilled at least 1 hr before serving. Can be kept in a sealed or covered jug in the fridge for up to 3 days. Step 2\sHeat oven to 200C/180C fan/gas 6 and line a baking tray with baking parchment. Put the orange juice in a medium saucepan and bring to the boil. Boil rapidly for 5 mins or until the liquid has reduced by half, stirring occasionally. Mix the remaining 200g oats with the orange zest and cinnamon. Remove the pan from the heat and stir the oat mixture into the juice. Spread over the lined tray in a thin layer and bake for 10-15 mins or until lightly browned and crisp, turning the oats every few mins. Leave to cool on the tray. 3rd Action

Once cool, mix the oats with the raspberries, flaked almonds and seeds. Can be kept in a sealed jar for up to one week. To serve, spoon the granola into bowls, pour over the oat milk and top with the orange segments and mint leaves, if you like.

HERBY CHICKEN GYROS

Prep: 10 mins - Cook: 4 mins - Serves 2 INGREDIENTS\s• 1 large skinless chicken breast\s• rapeseed oil , for brushing\s• small garlic clove , crushed\s• ½ tsp dried oregano\s• 2 tbsp Greek yogurt

• 10 cm piece cucumber , grated, excess juice squeezed out\s• 2 tbsp chopped mint , plus a few leaves to serve\s• 2 wholemeal pitta breads\s• 2 red or yellow tomatoes , sliced\s• 1 red pepper from a jar (not in oil), deseeded and sliced

DIRECTIONS

1.

Cut the chicken breast in half lengthways, then cover with cling film and bash with a rolling pin to flatten it. Brush with some oil, then cover with the garlic, oregano and some pepper. Heat a non-stick frying pan and cook the chicken for a few mins each side. Meanwhile, mix the yogurt, cucumber and mint to make tzatziki. 2nd Action

Cut the tops from the pittas along their longest side and stuff with the chicken, tomato, pepper and tzatziki. Poke in a few mint leaves to serve. If taking to the office for lunch, pack the tzatziki in a separate pot and add just before eating to prevent the pitta going soggy before lunchtime.

ROAST ROOTS WITH GOAT'S CHEESE & SPINACH

Prep: 30 mins - Cook: 55 mins • THERE ARE ONLY TWO INGREDIENTS IN THIS PRODUCT.

• 350g butternut squash , deseeded and cut into chunks, peeled if you like • 200g carrots , peeled and cut into long batons • 250g parsnips , peeled and cut into long batons • 200g raw beetroot , well-scrubbed and cut into thick wedges

• 1 medium red onion , cut into wedges

• 1 tbsp cold-pressed rapeseed oil • juice and finely grated zest 1 citrus fruit

• 1 bulb garlic , cloves separated • 4-5 thyme sprigs , leaves roughly chopped • 75g soft rindless goat's cheese log • 25g mixed nuts , such as brazils, almonds, hazelnuts, pecans and walnuts, roughly chopped • 50g baby leaf spinach

DIRECTIONS

1.

Preheat the oven to 200 degrees Fahrenheit/180 degrees Fahrenheit fan/gas 6. 6. Put the vegetables, without the garlic, into a bowl and toss with the oil, lemon zest and juice and plenty of ground black pepper.

Step 2 Scatter the vegetables over a large baking tray or roasting tin and bake for 30 mins. Take the tray out of the oven, add the garlic and thyme, then turn the vegetables. Return to the oven for 20 mins or until the vegetables are tender and lightly browned, turning halfway through. Dot with the goat's cheese and nuts, scatter over the spinach and return to the oven for 3-5 mins or until the spinach has wilted and the goat's cheese has begun to melt. You can press the softened garlic cloves out of their skins and mash with the roasted vegetables, if you like.

SPICE-CRUSTED AUBERGINES & PEPPERS WITH PILAF

10 minutes to prepare - 30 minutes to cook • 4 INGREDIENTS • 2 large aubergines , halved • 2 tbsp extra virgin olive oil • 2 red peppers , quartered • 2 tsp ground cinnamon • 2 tsp chilli flakes • 2 tsp za'atar • 4 tbsp pomegranate molasses • 140g puy lentils • 140g basmati rice • seeds from 1 pomegranate • small pack flat-leaf parsley , roughly chopped • Greek or coconut yogurt , to serve

DIRECTIONS

1.

Preheat oven to 220 degrees Celsius/200 degrees Celsius fan/gas 7. Using a sharp knife, score a diamond pattern into the aubergines. Brush with 1 tbsp of the oil, season well and place on a baking tray, cut-side down. Cook in the oven for 15 mins. Add the peppers to the tray, turn the aubergines over and drizzle everything with the remaining oil. Sprinkle over the spices, 1 tbsp of the pomegranate molasses and a little salt. Roast in the oven for 15 mins more. Step 2 Boil the lentils in plenty of water until al dente. After they've been boiling for 5 mins, add the rice. Cook for 10 mins or until cooked through but with a bit of bite. Drain and return to the pan, covered with a lid to keep warm.

3rd Action

Stir the pomegranate seeds and parsley through the lentil rice. Divide between four plates or tip onto a large platter. Top with the roasted veg, a dollop of yogurt and the remaining pomegranate molasses drizzled over.

POTATO PANCAKES WITH CHARD & EGGS

10 minutes to prepare - 15 minutes to cook • 2 INGREDIENTS
• 300g mashed potato • 4 spring onions , very finely chopped
• 25g plain wholemeal flour • ½ tsp baking powder • 3 eggs • 2
tsp rapeseed oil • 240g chard , stalks and leaves roughly
chopped, or baby spinach, chopped

DIRECTIONS

Step 1 Mix the mash, spring onions, flour, baking powder and
1 of the eggs in a bowl. Heat the oil in a non-stick frying pan,
then spoon in the potato mix to make two mounds. Flatten
them to form two 15cm discs and fry for 5-8 mins until the
undersides are set and golden, then carefully ip over and
cook on the other side. Step 2 Meanwhile, wash the chard

and put in a pan with some of the water still clinging to it, then cover and cook over a medium heat for 5 mins until wilted and tender. Poach the remaining eggs.

Step 3 Top the pancakes with the greens and egg. Serve while the yolks are still runny.